Monographs on Endocrinology

Volume 11

Edited by

F. Gross, Heidelberg · A. Labhard, Zürich · M. B. Lipsett, Cleveland
T. Mann, Cambridge · L. T. Samuels (†), Salt Lake City
J. Zander, München

Susumu Ohno

Major Sex-Determining Genes

With 34 Figures

Springer-Verlag Berlin · Heidelberg · New York 1979

Dr. Susumu Ohno

Department of Biology
City of Hope
National Medical Center
1500 East Duarte Road
California-USA

ISBN 3-540-08965-9 Springer-Verlag Berlin Heidelberg NewYork
ISBN 0-387-08965-9 Springer Verlag NewYork Heidelberg Berlin

Library of Congress Cataloging in Publication Data

Ohno, Susumu. Major sex determining genes. (Monographs on endocrinology; v. 11) Bibliography: p. includes index. 1. Sex-Cause and determination. 2. Sexual dimorphism (Animals) 3. Gene expression. 4. Sex chromosomes. 5. Mammals-Physiology. I. Title. [DNLM: 1. Sex determination. 2. Sex chromosomes. 3. Genes. WI MO57 v. 11 / QH600.5 038m]
QP251.037 599'.01'6 78-10285

Printed in Germany

Typesetting: R. Leipe, Hagenbach, Germany
Printing and binding: Brandstetter, Wiesbaden, Germany
2125/3020 - 543210

To Midori

in anticipation of our coming silver wedding anniversary

Preface

Upon wresting the control of the earth from the Titans, Zeus assigned the task of creating living creatures to two Titan brothers who had sided with him in the epic battle just concluded. Because Epimetheus, who had been endowed only with hindsight, had the first hand in this creation, all the good attributes were exhausted by the time the lion, the elephant and other animals were created. When the time came for the creation of man, there were precious few materials left to work with. Not surprisingly, man was made weak and naked. Prometheus took pity on this miscreation and gave man the use of fire. For this foresight, Zeus meted out horrible punishment, binding Prometheus to a rocky pillar in the Caucasas Mountains and letting a vulture consume his liver daily.

It seems to me that the ancient Greeks in their unfathomable wisdom understood the essence of the evolutionary process very well. Had Escherichia coli of 200 million years or so ago been endowed with the foresight to anticipate the eventual emergence of and subsequent dominance by mammals of this Earth, they would no doubt have equipped themselves, in anticipation of the coming certainty, with the lac operon to deal with lactose in the suckling mammalian infant's gut. Had they been able to do so, the actual emergance of mammals would have exerted no selective pressure upon existing E. COLI. In this manner, we come to realize that foresight is forbidden and that only hindsight prevails in the Darwinian world of evolution by natural selection. Today, it is becoming fashionable to believe in the rigid heritability of human intelligence. If our intelligence too is the product of natural selection, the lack of foresight must be inherent in our intelligence.

In 1967, I published my first monograph, *Sex Chrosmosomes and Sex-Linked Genes*, as the first of this very series by the same publisher. There was already a great deal to discuss concerning the dosage compensation mechanism for X-linked genes caused by random X-inactivation in the female, and the evolutionary conservation in toto of the mammalian X-linkage group. Unfortunately, the sex-linked genes then under discussion had nothing whatsoever to do with the mammalian sex-determining mechanism *per se*. For this central theme, there was precious little to talk about. Indeed, we have come a long way in the last ten years. Yet, looking back, I am appalled by my own lack of foresight. After all, H-Y antigen became known in 1955. Furthermore, its discoverer, E. J. Eichwald, spent a few months in my laboratory during the early 1960s. Although I have a suspicion that Eichwald himself already suspected the possible role of his H-Y antigen in mammalian sex determination, I must admit that such a thought never crossed my mind at that time. Similarly, the testicular feminization syndrome of man had already become a well-defined entity in 1953. Yet I then regarded it merely as one of the multitude of structural mutations that cause all sorts of pseudohermaphrodisms and intersexualities. Accurcd is the human intelligence, bound by the hindsight of natural selection.

Acknowledgments

In chronological order, postdoctorate fellows of my laboratory during the last eight years were: R. Dofoku, U. Tettenborn, H. Itakura, S.R. Blecher, U. Drews, B. Attardi, K.C. Reed, Y. Nagai, and S. Ciccarese. Graduate and undergraduate students of the same period were D.A. Owen, L.N. Geller, T. Baruch, D. Stapleton, B. Beutler, H. Mitz, and R. Smith. Their contributions as well as the technical help of C. Stenius, G. Schipmann, N. Lee, L.C. Christian, M. Carter-Romero, E. Hodge, and C. Ivery are gratefuily acknowledged, and so is the financial support received from NIH contract NO1-CB-33907 and grants HD-CA-07975 and 1 RO1-AG-00042 as well as from the Bixby foundation.

I am also very grateful for intellectual stimuli provided by and cooperation received from my colleagues and good friends: C.W. Bardin, B.M. Cattanach, W. Engel, K.Fredga, A. Gropp, G. Klein, M.F. Lyon, G. Moller, R.V. Short, and U. Wolf. In addition, I owe special thanks to E.A. Boyse and S.S.Wachtel, who very kindly enticed me into the H-Y antigen immunology. Naturally, I should also likc to thank my secretary, N. L. Busse. My intellectual indebtedness in immunology to N.K. Jerne, and M. Cohn is also gratefully acknowledged.

Contents

Part I

Sexual Dimorphism as a Dispensable Appendage of the Sex-Determining Mechanism

Chapter 1

Why Sexual Dimorphism?

At the zoo, even a child has no difficulty in singling out a lion from his pride of lionesses. The king of beasts is not only endowed with his tell-tale mane, but is also conspicuously larger and more powerfully built than his female partners (Fig. 1). The same, however, does not hold true for the king and queen of winged creatures, for even a zoo expert has no certain way of distinguishing a male eagle from a female eagle (Fig. 2). In all parts of the world, these magnificent birds of prey are in danger of becoming extinct; accordingly, many zoos are attempting to breed them in captivity. The absolute lack of sexual dimorphism among many species of eagles has hindered these attempts, for there is an even chance that a breeding cage (established with considerable expense) contains a like-sexed pair. During the past few years, I have occasionally been consulted to determine the sex of individual eagles either by sex chromosome analysis or by H-Y antigen typing.

The foregoing contrast serves to illustrate that to be a successful hunter, a species need not manifest sexual dimorphism. In fact, most of the hunting is done by lionesses, while the king of beasts is not beyond stealing a carcass that a pack of hyenas has just brought down. Hyenas, on the other hand, are a rather exceptional mammalian species in that sexual dimorphism is not at all evident. The peculiar

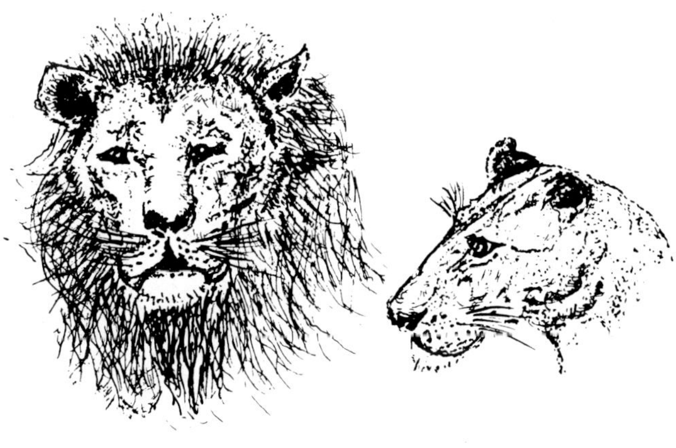

Fig. 1. A very pronounced sexual dimorphism illustrated by a mature lion and a young lioness of his harem. An old lion is purposely drawn in a slightly anthropomorphic manner to suggest a battle-worn king. There is little doubt that warriors of old identified themselves with males of other sexually dimorphic mammalian species. The stag's antlers, the bull's horns frequently adorned their war helmets. As to lions, one immediately recalls Richard *Coeur de Lion* of the third crusade, one of the several outstanding warrior kings of the Plantagenet line. In Germany, there was Henry the Lion of Brunswick, who rashly challenged the might of Frederick Barbarossa, the Holy Roman Emperor

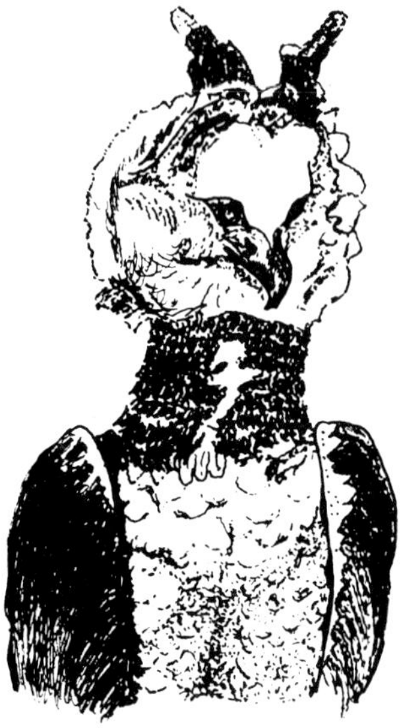

Fig. 2. A fierce harpy eagle (Harpia harpyja) of Central and South America. A decorative long crest and frill that covers the back of its neck is reminiscent of the lion's mane. Yet being sexually monomorphic, such decorative ornaments are worn by males and females alike. Although falconers in the king's retinue knowingly trained larger female falcons, if the sexual monomorphism and even occasional female supremacy among birds of prey had been common knowledge, I doubt if Roman legions as well as Napoleon's grand army would have marched under the eagle standards, for the eagle was no doubt thought of as another masculine supremacy symbol

clitorial enlargement of the female diminishes sexual dimorphism even with regard to the outward appearance of their genitalia. Yet hyenas are apparently as successful at hunting as at scavenging (LAWICK-GOODALL and LAWICK-GOODALL, 1970).

DARWIN (1871) himself realized that sexually dimorphic species tend to practice polygamous matings whereas the monomorphic ones tend to be a monogamous species; this generalization is essentially correct with regard to the example just mentioned. The large body size that characterizes many long-living mammalian species is invariably associated with long gestation periods and small litter size – often only one. Thus, the reproductive capacity of a population is determined by the number of breeding females it contains. A population can ill afford to reduce the number of these precious females by subjecting them to too intense a selective pressure. Furthermore, since she produces so few progeny in her lifetime, the extent of genetic contribution any individual female makes to the next generation of a population is quite limited. The one-to-one sex ratio in the above circumstance creates a great surplus of males that are readily dispensable. Inasmuch as a single male is capable of fertilizing a large number of females, if an intense intrasexual competition for the possession of females is elicited among males, the next generation of a population can be stamped with large genetic imprints of a few select males that emerged victorious. In this way, large mamalian species can compensate for, or even overcome the evolutionary slow-down caused by a long gestation period as well as a long generation time and a small litter size. Indeed, man has long utilized the principle of foundation sires to create desired breeds of domestic animals. In the mounted condition, English thoroughbred horses of today can sustain a speed of 38 mph for a mile or two. There is no swifter animal, wild or domestic. Yet this marvelous breed was created within a short span of 50 to 60 years starting from three Arabian and Barb stallions imported to England at the beginning of the eighteenth century. By 1764, the true foundation sire, Eclipse, was born.

Not surprisingly, a majority of large mammals is said to practice polygamous mating of the polygynous (many females) type (WILSON, 1975) and in these species, DARWIN was right in associating pronounced sexual dimorphism with polygamy. The polyandrous (many males) type of polygamy is of theoretical interest only, for it is impracticable for most mammalian species.

The problem begins whenever an attempt is made to extend this association between pronounced sexual dimorphism and polygamy to cover small mammals and animals of other classes. First of all, small mammals, as a rule, are characterized by short gestation periods and generation times as well as by large litter sizes. In this condition, females are not as indispensable as in the previous condition and a species can evolve with a reasonable rate without the benefit of polygamy. Furthermore, their behavior tends to depend more on olfactory cues than on visual ones. For example the mouse (Mus musculus) is clearly a polygamous species despite its miniscule size. Accordingly, males readily combat each other, even in a laboratory environment. Yet sexual dimorphism in this species is not obvious to our naked eyes and after repeated pregnancies, females actually grow larger than males. This apparent paradox is resolved when one realizes that intrasexual competition among male mice is elicited almost entirely by olfactory cues. A mature male mouse emits a particular body odor that provokes aggression from other males (MUGFORD and NOWELL, 1970), and he also marks his den with urinary pheromones that retard aggression of an intruder (JONES and NOWELL, 1974). Thus, being a resident, he gains a combative advantage over an intruder. These two types of pheromones are no doubt, very important ingredients in making the mouse not only a polygamous species, but also a highly territorial one.

In sharp contrast to mammals, a majority of avian species are said to be monogamous. The extensive modification of the basic vertebrate anatomy that enabled many species of birds to become swift and long-range flyers cannot readily be sacrificied for the sake of sexual dimorphism: Only a sexual difference in plumage coloring does not hinder their flying capacity. Intrasexual combats are likely to damage flight feathers of the victor as well as of the vanquished. To satisfy their high rate of metabolism and to compensate for their short intestine, birds consume a large amount of food disproportionate to their light body weight. Accordingly, during her attempt to hatch a clutch of eggs, a female faces the ugly prospect of starving to death. Even after a successful hatching of the eggs, the female, so weakened, is hard pressed to bring home sufficient food supplies to satisfy the voracious appetites of her hatched young. All of these conditions obviously call for the practice of monogamy that entails male-female cooperation in the rearing of the young. Yet, polygamy is still practices by some of the more sedentary, basically ground-living birds to whom flights are of secondary importance. Indeed, a very pronounced sexual dimorphism is encountered in the chicken, the pheasant, and the peacock, their males being endowed with very vivid plumage an obvious symbol of masculine supremacy. Anyone who has witnessed a cock fight, elaborately staged as a barbarous, but very ancient form of sporting event, should be deeply impressed by the intensity of the combative urge that one cock displays toward the other. Wild pheasant cocks, if vanquished in combat and therefore deprived of their harems, appear literally to shrink with disappointment and shame, and the old adage "dressed like a peacock" attests to the extreme of sexual dimorphism seen in this particular species of ground-living birds.

Nevertheless, the fact that a great majority of birds are of monogamous and often sexually monomorphic species appears to have had something to do with the not very impressive adaptive radiations exhibited by members of the class *Aves*. There is considerable justification in calling birds glorified reptiles and the overall karyologic conservatism displayed by birds is in sharp contrast to the daring display of karyologic diversities exhibited by mammalian species. There is little doubt that the manifestation of sexual dimorphism and the ensuing practice of polygynous matings contributed greatly to the spectacular evolutionary success of mammals.

Chapter 2

Man as a Sexually Dimorphic Species

Sexual dimorphism is quite pronounced in two of the three closest relatives of man: gorillas and orangutans. Males are noticeably larger and more powerfully built than females and a few masculine display characteristics are also evident: i.e., large canine teeth. Indeed, they are said to be the practitioners of polygamy, although befitting their intelligence, the practice is said to be quite subtle in that a dominant male manages to placate subordinate males by allowing them to copulate with females in heat when these females are either at the beginning or at the end of estrus, so that while they are receptive to males, they are in no danger of being impregnated. While sexual dimorphism became less obvious in chimpanzees, it became very pronounced once again in man. Mature males, if left unshaven, grow luxuriant beards and the penis and scrotum are extraordinarily conspicuous and large, suggesting that they are not merely for reproductive function but that they once served as a symbolic display of masculine supremacy. The abundant use of phallic symbols by many cultures appears to substantiate this idea. Although the practice of polygynous matings has apparently been uncommon in human history, the inclination to do so appears to have always been there; notice the inclusion of such words as "harem" and "seraglio", or their equivalents, in human vocabularies. Those human genes awakened at puberty by androgens, must have been whispering to the ears of the sexually mature man that he ought to behave as bulls or lions do. It has been observed that when a rival lion takes over a pride of lionesses, the first royal decree issued is often to kill off the youngest cubs (BERTRAM, 1975). By so doing, the male has eliminated the progeny of his supplanted rivals and has speeded up the female s return to estrus and hence the first opportunity to propagate his own seeds.

William Shakespeare, who apparently adopted the twisted view of Tudor historians about the last Plantagenet, attributes nearly all the deeds of the lion noted above to King Richard III. Rivals and the progeny of rivals he had reputedly slain include the Lancastrian heir, Edward, his brother George, Duke of Clarence, as well as his kingly brother's two sons: Edward V and Richard, Duke of York. He first possessed Anne, the bride of the first-named Edward, then wooed Elizabeth, the daughter of Edward IV and the sister of his two infant victims.

There apparently are many justifications in seeking the cause of warfare in combative urges of human males that are induced by the postpubertal androgen activation of a specific set of genes (OHNO, 1976a). Helmets and suits of armor, with which knights and samurais alike engaged in their mortal combats, were often so decorative and elaborate that they must have seriously hindered their combative efficiencies. One is immediately reminded of the massive antlers of the great Irish stag (Megaceros gigantus) that may have caused the extinction of that species (SHORT, 1976). Were it not for the destructive power of modern firearms, the officers' uniforms of today's field armies also would likely have remained as colorful as the plumage of peacocks. The above being the case, should one view incessant warfare in human histories as the just manifestation of the sound evolutionary strategy universally adapted by sexually dimorphic mammalian species? An attempt to justify wars on evolutionary grounds was actually made in 1911, by General Friedrich VON BERNHARDI (1914). Perhaps he should be regarded as the founding father of human sociobiology. Upon winning victories, human male combatants often exterminated rival mature males and enslaved women and children, as the Athenians did on the island of Mellos during the Peloponnesian Wars, and as so many others have done on countless occasions. Occasionally, the even more extreme measure of complete extermination was carried out, as Edward the Black Prince did to the inhabitants of Limoges. These acts also can be regarded as a logical extension of the basic evolutionary strategy of a sexually dimorphic species.

Although many of our generation still have a living memory of the agelong glorification of armed conflicts, it is likely that today's readers of this article will unanimously regard the human masculine behaviors, noted above as particularly base and obnoxious. The ascent of man through the ages of cicilization has been phenomenally rapid in the time scale of evolution. For this rise, within at the most 10,000 years, genetic changes can claim no credit, for evolution by natural selection is an agonizingly slow process especially for long-living mammals of large body size such as man. The exact amino acid sequence identity found in many proteins of man and the chimpanzee verifies the slowness of Darwinian evolution as it operates among advanced primates (KING and WILSON, 1975).

It would appear that man's gradual realization of the futility of unbridled masculine behavior played no small part in his rapid ascent through the ages of civilization. Obviously, it is not easy, to ignore specific dictates of his genomes. The recurrent theme of conflict between the soul and bodily desires in the great writings of the past attests to the difficulties involved in transforming the above realization into actual deeds. Nevertheless, it seems to me that the very invention of such terms as "soul" and "spirit" reflects the importance that man came to attach to the necessity of suppressing certain specific manifestations of the sexually mature males' androgen-induced gene activities. Despite being a very sexually dimorphic species, our species clearly owes its evolutionary success, based on extraordinary intelligence, to the practice of monogamy. Only the stable male-female pair bond can accommodate the characteristically slow growth of human infants, and the subsequent period of long apprenticeship that juveniles go through while under parental care, which is essential to the nurturing of their native intelligence as well as to assimilation of the knowledge that their predecessors have accumulated. When in the evolutionary development of man did this drastic switch from the polygynous mating system befitting a very sexually dimorphic species, to the monogamous mating system normally associated with a sexually monomorphic species take place: and what was the motivating factor primarily responsible for this switch?

It is thought that as the Earth began to cool off during early Pliocene times (10 million years or so ago), brachiating apes of that time faced two alternatives: to retreat with receding forests as the ancestors of the chimpanzees and gorillas apparently did, or to stay in the emerging savanna to try out a new way of life as hunting apes, as our ancestors are thought to have done (MORRIS, 1967). This then was clearly the time to reform the polygynous mating system. As neophyte hunters, their individual hunting prowess must have been dismal. In order to feed upon large ungulates of the savanna, while themselves not falling victims to large carnivores, they must have had no choice but to adapt the hunting-by-a-pack method as practiced by hyenas, African wild dogs, and wolves. One could hardly expect subordinate males, deprived of females, to be willing participants in a hunting pack. The recruitment of all available adult males to a hunting pack ist clearly more compatible with the monogamous mating system. To meet this new requirement in social organization, one might have thought natural selection to begin favoring the development of sexual monomorphism by progressive curtailment of the manifestation of masculine supremacy symbols in adult males. Yet many of the symbols of masculine supremacy with which today's adult human males are adorned are clearly not the evolutionary carryovers from his pre-Pliocene days, because these symbols are uniquely human as already noted. Accordingly, they are very different from those of male chimpanzees and gorillas, the two closest living relatives of man.

The virtual absence of sexual dimorphism in hyenas apparently reflects the nearly equal hunting prowess between the sexes. Not surprisingly, matriarchal clans are found among hyenas (LAWICK-GOODALL and LAWICK-GOODALL, 1970). For the human ancestors, by contrast, it appears that hunting in packs, from its start, became a more or less adult male-specific occupation. With the decision to remain in the emerging savanna, our brachiating ape ancestors did not become carnivorous but rather omnivorous, as our teeth which are still better fit for the grinding of grains and leaves than for the tearing of meat, testify. Gathering supplies of plant food appeared to become the task of adult females and juveniles. This division of labor between the sexes was obviously conducive to the further development of intelligence by man's ape ancestors. The full participation of adult females in a hunting pack would have mitigated against a very important initiation of an evolutionary trend toward progressive prolongation of the infantile growth period, for its prerequisite is the adult female's devotion to the care of her infants. Without this prolongation, a phenomenal rise in man's intellectual capacity would not have begun.

I believe that the foregoing is the evolutionary reason for the preservation and even continuous accentuation of sexual dimorphism that has accompanied the emergence of man despite the abandoned practice of polygynous matings. Not only was the preservation of sexual difference in body size and muscular strength conducive to the previously described division of labor, but also the illusion of masculine supremacy, enhanced by conspicuous biological symbols, must have furnished the necessary motivation for sexually mature males to engage in hazardous tasks of hunting down large ungulates of great strength.

It would appear that a switch from the polygamous to monogamous mating system by human ancestors was accomplished without genetically curtailing the male's propensity toward combativeness and polygamy. In most mammalian species, the attractiveness of females to males undergoes cyclical variations reaching its height at the time of the female's estrus. Thus, males are afforded with periodic respites from the all-consuming urge to reproduce. What if adult females became attractive to males every day of the year? I would rather think that, under the circumstances, even the prowess of the most dominant of the inherently polygynous males would be overmatched and proven inadequate to satisfy the needs of the multitude of females in his harem. In this way, inherently polygynous males may be enticed to start favoring the monogamous mating system. This, in fact, appears to have been the exact evolutionary strategy adapted by female members of man's ancestors. Indeed, an adult woman's mammary glands are no longer the mere organ of lactation, rather a pair of well-shaped breasts, conspicuous without the benefit of pregnancy and ensuing lactation, serve as a constant reminder of feminine attractiveness, and human females are constantly receptive to the male's copulatory urge except for monthly periods of menses (MORRIS, 1967).

Probably because of the sexual division of labor noted above, a switch from the polygynous to the monogamous mating system was accomplished, not by abolishing preexisting sexual dimorphism, but rather by adding female-specific postpubertal developments to greatly enhance sexual dimorphism. Herein apparently was laid the seed of phenomenal success that man, as a species, subsequently enjoyed as well as of the potential disaster that looms in our future. The inherent combativeness among human males obviously harks back to the day of polygamy. Whether one likes it or not, there is no denying that, until the end of the last great World War, the history of mankind had largely been shaped by successions of armed conflicts. In the feudal society, armed conflicts preferentially involved members of the warrior class. This makes good biological sense indeed for this class was nonproductive in that it did not contribute either agricultural products or artifacts to the society. Thus, there again was a great surplus of males peculiar to this class, which made intense intrasexual selection again practicable. Was it this selection that elevated victorious warriors as lords in all feudal societies of the past? Needless to say, the vast destruction of material resources and the indiscriminate killing of women and juveniles that modern wars entail totally abolished whatever evolutionary justification human warfare might have had when it was practiced among surplus males of the warrior class. The ultimate fate of man as a species appears to depend upon the degree of success that man achieves in either curtailing or diverting the ancient combative urges of adult males.

Chapter 3

Male Chauvinism and a Misunderstanding of Sexual Dimorphism

As a species, man is a study in contradictions. Having evolved as brachiating apes in pre-Pliocene forests, he tried a new way of life in the emerging savanna as a hunting ape and succeeded in becoming omnivorous. Yet his teeth are still designed for the grinding of grains and leaves only, and ill-fit for the seizing of prey. While retaining and even accentuating sexual dimorphism, he abandoned the practice of polygynous matings and became monogamous. In the humid heat of pre-Pliocene forests, he was a hairy ape. Yet he became a "naked ape" prior to his territorial expansion to the temperate zone with cold winters. Because of a congenital deficiency in *de novo* synthesis of vitamin C, men of the temperate zone used to suffer through long winters for the want of fresh fruits. Such contradictions are abundantly evident in human behavior as well. Institutionalized followers of the Man who preached to turn the other cheek, tortured and burned fellow beings by branding them as heretics. Knowing the total futility of infantry charges against an entrenched nest of machine guns, those charges were repeated all the same throughout the First World War, causing the loss of millions in the flower of their youth.

Yet we must owe progressive refinements of our intelligence to such evolutionary contradictions that created endless inner conflicts within the soul of man. Comparing the average rate of amino acid substitutions per gene product with the rate of progressive extension of the longevity during the course of primate evolution, it has been convincingly argued that the number of gene loci involved in giving extraordinary longevity to man must necessarily be very small (CUTLER, 1974). Knowing the already noted near genetic identity between man and the chimpanzee, his closest living relative (KING and WILSON, 1975), the same convincing sort of argument can be made to suggest that species-specific differences, at only tens of gene loci, separate human intelligence from that of chimpanzees. Because it now appears that, until a few years ago, man had grossly underestimated the intelligence of chimpanzees (GARDNER and GARDNER, 1975), such an argument is quite plausible. As already noted, natural selection can claim no credit to the phenomenally rapid ascent of man through the ages of civilization. The native intelligence of man that has not improved during the last 10,000 years might indeed be only a little better than that of chimpanzees. The social or cultural evolution of the last 10,000 years that elevated club-yielding savages to men of culture may indeed be due to progressively successful exploitation of rather meager genetic resources.

I would not be surprised if the motivating force of human cultural evolution is identified as man's inner conflicts brought about by various evolutionary contradictions inherent in our species. Without such inner conflicts, how can man conceive of the soul as the controlling element of his bodily desires. The objectivity in appraising a given event was apparently born when man learned to be a third-party observer of an event, regardless of whether or not he is a participant in it. Without developing the concept of "soul", could man be a participant and an observer at the same time?

To my mind, Athenians living during the time of the Peloponnesian Wars, were one of the most civilized peoples in all of human history. Yet the men's attitude toward women was no more enlightened than that of any other society. Legitimate wives were thought of as an instrument for propagating their seeds. While there were women of questionable virtue to gratify their sexual desires, true love was apparently reserved for homosexual relationships with male youths. To me there is no better testimony to the long-rooted biological basis of male chauvinism. Were we to be as sexually monomorphic as eagles or hyenas, the notion of male chauvinism would never have entered the mind of man. Obviously what is to blame is the fact of being a sexually dimorphic species as well as the adult male's genetic memory of the past practice of polygynous matings. Were we to accept the currently popular notion that the genes in our genome make us behave the way we do (DAWKINS, 1976), we should accept male chauvinism as a fact of human life. Yet such acceptance is no better than that of incessant warfare as a fact of life. Since both practices are rooted in the same cause, were we to curtail one so should we the other.

Furthermore, the grandiose notion of masculine supremacy has a way of blinding even competent biologists provided that they are men. Thus, one often hears the statement that men and women are so genetically different that they might as well be regarded as two different species. Nothing is further from the truth, yet the notion of a battle between the sexes as an evolutionary process is based on this nonsense.

Man applies but one specific selective pressure for ever higher yields of milk upon the Holstein-Friesian breed of cattle. Yet this uniquely female trait has been markedly improved by the use of progressively smaller numbers of stud bulls of the highest quality through artificial insemination. Men in time even learned to dentify the exemplary phenotype of the Holstein bull that is likely to sire daughters who are prodigious milk producers. While these exemplary Holstein bulls are no match in combative prowess to Spanish fighting bulls, they have neither enlarged udders nor an exceptionally wide pelvic girdle. They are impressively masculine in their ponderous way.

While there are fighting cocks, there are no fighting hens, for the combative urge is unique to males of the polygynous species. Yet a successful breeder of fighting cocks pays as much attention to the genetic background and phenotype of hens as to those of cocks in his breeding stock. In time, he learns, to identify the exemplary phenotype of hens that is likely to produce future champion fighting cocks, and these hens will not look like fighting cocks. Thus, we come to realize that in order to reap evolutionary benefits from the practice of polygynous matings, genetic differences between the sexes should be kept at a necessary minimum so that heritable traits, selected as a result of intense combative competitions among adult males, shall benefit male and female progeny alike of the next generation. To do so, the expression of these selected traits, if they are sex specific, should come under the control of sex steroid hormones to avoid the manifestation of masculine traits by female progeny. Indeed, aside from the male-specific Y chromosome, there are no meaningful sexual differences in the genetic constitution of mammalian species. Disparity in the number of X chromosomes is minimized by the X-inactivation mechanism (LYON, 1961; BEUTLER, et al., 1962). In almost all the somatic cells of a female's body, only one or the other X chromosome functions. With regard to the Y chromosome, unlike other chromosomes that are endowed with thousands of divergent genes, this male-specific chromosome is a genetic dummy knowing but one function. All the biological symbols of masculine supremacy are not the reflection of male-specific genes, but they are the traits induced by a male steroid hormone – testosterone. As such, all these symbols can be readily induced on females by persistent administration of androgen throughout the fetal and postpubertal life. Sexual dimorphism, secondarily induced by sex steroid hormones, is but a dispensable appendage of the basic sex-determining mechanism shared in common by all the mammalian species, sexually dimorphic as well as monomorphic species.

We have thus seen the first of the several apparent evolutionary paradoxes to be encountered in this book. Only because the mammalian sex-determining mechanism is founded on the principle that a genetic disparity between two sexes shall be kept at the absolute minimum required for bisexual reproduction, a majority of the mammalian species have been able to derive substantial evolutionary benefits from the manifestation of very pronounced sexual dimorphism and the consequent practice of polygynous matings.

Part II

H-Y Antigen and Chromosomal Determination of Primary (Gonadal) Sex

Chapter 4

The Number of Genes in the Mammalian Genome and the Need for Master Regulatory Genes

The genome size (the amount of DNA contained in the haploid set of chromosomes) is fairly uniform among divergent mammalian species. It consists characteristically of about 3 x 10^9 DNA base pairs, thus the mammalian genome is roughly 1000 times the size of the Escherichia coli genome. Any notion of proportionality between the degree of the organism's complexity and the genome size, however, should quickly be dispelled by the realization that a sluggish lungfish, Lepidosiren paradoxa, is endowed with a genome 35 times greater than that of mammals (OHNO and ATKIN, 1966). In fact, such unyieldingly enormous genomes characterize crossopterygian lungfish as well as tailed amphibians, e.g., salamanders and newts. Among flowering plants too, one finds, a peculiar situation with regard to the genome size. For example, four species belonging to the genus Lathyrus are apparently endowed with the identical karyotype as far as the chromosome number and morphology are concerned ($2n=14$). Yet there is a maximum difference of threefold in their genome sizes (REES, 1972). Although life on this Earth owes its existence to the capacity of DNA to semiconservatively replicate itself, based on the inherent complementarity that exists between two pairs of bases, it would appear that a part in which functional messages are encoded constitutes a third or less of the eukaryotic genomic DNA.

At this point, it might be of interest to recall what only several years ago was considered to be a reasonable argument. The argument developed along the following line: A polypeptide chain, 300 amino acid residues long, may be considered as the average size of multitudes of the polypeptide chains synthesized by mammalian cells. Since each amino acid in the peptide chain is specified by three consecutive bases (triplet codons), the average size of mammalian genes should then be about 1000 base pairs long. Accordingly, the mammalian genome has room for three million genes.

Germ-line theorists on the origin of antibody diversities used to find the above argument particularly attractive. Inasmuch as each individual mammal is capable of generating tens of thousands of antibodies directed against wide varieties of naturally occurring as well as man-made antigens, it was argued that the mammalian genome might be endowed with half a million or so genes for immunoglobulin light and heavy-chain variable regions. In view of the important role that the immune defense system plays in the well-being of mammalian individuals, to devote one-sixth of the total number of genes for this purpose appeared not all together unreasonable. Nucleic acid hybridization experiments, utilizing C-DNA copies of monoclonal myeloma immunoglobulin light-chain *messenger* RNAs, however, have subsequently shown that the actual number of variable-region genes that the mammalian genome harbors is quite small (e.g.) HOZUMI and TONEGAWA,

1976). The idea that antibody diversities are generated mainly by somatic mutations of a relatively small number of variable-region genes appears to have finally been vindicated (e.g. JERNE, 1971). Today, even germ-line theorists are content with only a few hundred immunoglobulin variable-region genes in the mammalian genome.

Among other things, the types of arguments for the existence of a few million genes in the mammalian genome have grossly underestimated the size of individual genes. Mammalian hemoglobin (Hb) -chain consists of 140 or 141 amino acid residues, whereas the Hb β-chain is 145 or 146 amino acid residues long. Even processed Hb *messenger* RNAs found in the cytoplasm, however, are already considerably greater in size than what many had expected them to be. The *messenger* RNAs consist of about 600 bases not counting the poly A tail at their 3' ends. Furthermore, it has recently been shown that nuclear precursors of these *messenger* RNAs (so-called heterogeneous nuclear RNAs) are as large as 27S in size (BASTOS and AVIV, 1977). Thus the hemoglobin α - as well as β-chain gene, which specifies a polypeptide chain of smaller than the average size, must itself be at least 5000 base pairs long. The average-sized mammalian gene specifying a 300 amino acid residue-long peptide chain might then be as long as 11,000 base pairs. It would appear that the mammalian genome has room to accommodate not three million genes but merely three hundred thousand genes. As to the actual number of genes, this revised figure appears still to be a gross overestimate, for individual genes on mammalian chromosomal DNA apparently are spaced rather widely apart by nontranscribed spacer sequences. The indication of the above can be found in the fact that the same genetic distance represents different physical distances in divergent organisms. In mammals, the genetic distance of one crossover unit covers roughly 10^6 base pairs, whereas the same genetic distance when applied to prokaryocytes merely represents 10^3 to 10^4 base pairs.

A gene can be defined as a stretch of DNA base sequences that contribute to the well-being of individual organisms either by specifying a product (ribosomal RNA, transfer RNA, or a polypeptide chain) or by functioning as a recognition signal to regulatory proteins (promotor or operator). Since the gene's assigned function is encoded in its DNA base sequence, its mutational alterations can cause the loss of its assigned function. Consequently, such mutations are deleterious to individuals who inherit them, and natural selection efficiently eliminates these unfit individuals and, therefore, these deleterious mutations. The fact that the histone IV (110 amino acid residues) of cattle and that of garden pea differ from each other by only two amino acid substitions (DELANGE and FAMBROUGH, 1968: MCLAUGHLIN and DAYHOFF, 1969) attests to the efficacy of natural selection. Natural selection has apparently managed to eliminate most of the mutations randomly sustained by this histone gene during the period of a billion years or so. It follows then that an organsim has to pay for the privilege of having each gene based on its probability of sustaining deleterious mutations.

Accordingly, an organism can exterminate itself by having too many genes in the genome, for its overall mutation load then becomes unbearable. The simple fact of life – that the spontaneous deleterious mutation rate per gene locus per organism's generation is of the order of 10^{-5} – thus, places a finite upper limit upon the number of gene loci any mammalian species can afford to maintain. Any stretch of DNA in which any and all mutational alterations are permissible, by definition, cannot have a specifically assigned function. There exists no obvious constraint against the accumulation by the genome of this kind of DNA. This may be the very reason why lungfish, salamanders, and newts came to posses extraordinarily enormous genomes. Needless to say, as the genome size increases, so does the cell size.

The total cell surface represented by a small number of large cells is considerably less than that by a large number of small cells. Accordingly, large cell size is incompatible with a metabolically active life. Yet, the very sluggish way of life led by lungfish and salamanders appears quite compatible with the large cell size, which is the consequence of having unyieldingly large genomes. In this manner, we come to realize one of the many striking paradoxes of evolution: A fraction of the genome that has been undergoing the fastest evolutionary changes is likely to represent the most trivial, and therefore, the most readily dispensable portion of the genomic DNA. On the contrary, real genes, those stretches of DNA that embody heritable messages, are to be found in the fraction that has been conserved in evolution to the extreme. At this point, however, we should recall the already noted fact that fresh transcripts (heterogenous nuclear RNAs) of mammalian genes are enormous in their sizes. Compared to compact prokaryotic genes, mammalian genes are quite untidy containing a number of noncoding base sequences within. Some of these noncoding sequences have been found as an insert within the coding region. For example, the DNA insert consisting of 550 base pairs has been found at the position corresponding to amino acids 104-105 of mouse hemoglobin β-chain. Since, this sequence, not found in the cytoplasmic messenger, was found in the 15S nuclear precursor (TILGHMAN et al, 1978), the same sequence has to be present in a larger 27S fresh transcript (BASTOS and AVIV, 1977). Many of the modern genes of higher vertebrates arose by the apparent fusion of two or more tandemly duplicated genes (OHNO, 1974). Inasmuch as the literal fusion of two coding regions requires the mechanical precision imposed by the triplet coding system, higher vertebrates apparently found it easier to transcribe two adjacent genes as one messenger RNA precursor and then developing the mean to clip off the transcribed spacer sequence between two adjacent coding regions; hence, the birth of a new gene which is tandem repeats of the old also gave rise to an insert. Thus, dispensable DNA base sequences are found not only between genes but also within individual genes of higher vertebrates. These dispensable DNA base sequences should be excluded from our consideration of the mutation load. From what was thought to be the observed overall deleterious mutation rate per human genome, CROW and KIMURA (1970) arrived at the figure of 4×10^4 as the total number of gene loci contained in the human genome. As stated on many previous occasions, I too believe the total number of gene loci that the mammalian genome harbors to be somewhat below one hundred thousand.

The gene loci numbering one hundred thousand is clearly more manageable than a few million gene loci, yet 10^5 is still a very large number, and the task of making them behave as a cohesive genomic unit by orchestrating their activities must be formidable. Indeed, it would appear that mammals do not always succeed in this attempt at orchestration. Recent advances in pharmacogenetics have substantiated the old proverb that one man's medicine is the other man's poison. Similarly, in multicellular organisms of the mammal's complexity, the situation may often arise in which a given mutation that is deleterious to one organ or one cell type is by chance beneficial to another organ or cell type. When the beneficiary is a germ cell, the consequence can be disastrous, for through better-fit germ cells, a deleterious mutation may propagate itself in a polulation. Wisely, mammals usually manage to suppress the haploid gene expression in their gametes, and this indeed is a very effective way of avoiding the type of disaster noted above. Nevertheless, minor disasters of these kinds are known to occur. For example, certain alleles of the T (tail-less) locus of the mouse are clearly deleterious, for even benign ones cause malformations of the vertebral column, whereas many are embryonic lethals. Yet their elimination from a population is made difficult by the fact that the male heterozygous for one of these alleles preferentially transmits that deleterious allele to his progeny (BRADEN, 1972).

As already noted, sexually dimorphic mammalian species tend to practice the polygynous mating system. Accordingly, males of these species engage in intense combative activities among each other for the possession of females. What if the combination of heritable traits that gives a decisive combative advantage to males, by making them more muscular and superaggressive, at the same time lowers their fertility? A mockery is then made of the polygynous mating system. Indeed, the mammalian genome is constantly hard pressed by contradictory demands made upon it. Males of sexually dimorphic species are often endowed with a combative weapon. Because it is used against other males of the same species, such a weapon tends to become more ornamental than lethal. If the old dominant male is given a lethal weapon, he will kill off all the young challengers in combat, many of them his sons, thus depriving himself of his heirs. Indeed, magnificent antlers of the stag, while impressively ornamental, are very inefficient as a combat weapon, and herein lies the problem. The other task assigned to the dominant male is the protection of his harem of adult females and juveniles from predators. Having been saddled with an ornamental weapon of doubtful combative value, the stag is rather delinquent in the performance of his assigned function as a protector. It appears that antlers grown too massively ornamental actually caused the extinction of the great Irish deer (Megaceros gigantus), as already noted (SHORT, 1976).

The preceding examples should suffice to make us realize the desperate need of the mammalian genome. The genes approaching one hundred thousand in number must somehow be organized into a cohesive unit. Only then can the genome have a chance of finding a succession of reasonable compromise solutions, most of the time in dealing with the contradictory demands constantly made upon it. Thus, these numerous genes cannot be left alone to go their separate ways. They should be controlled by successive series of genetic regulatory systems that constitute an orderly hierarchy. This regulatory orderliness, I believe, is the hallmark of mammals (OHNO, 1976b).

If viewed from the bottom, any mammalian genetic regulatory system is bound to appear very complicated, for it consists of a very large number of structural genes. Furthermore, these structural genes are no doubt partitioned into a set of subsidiary regulatory systems, and the individual structural genes are often placed under dual controls, because the same structural gene may belong to two or more different regulatory systems. Yet all of these often overlapping subsidiary regulatory systems must eventually come unter the control of one or the other of a small number of master regulatory genes

The above was the very reason for my statement of some years ago that if viewed from the top of a given heirarchy, each mammalian genetic regulatory system should reveal itself to be simple and straightforward (OHNO, 1971). Indeed, the mammalian sex-determining mechanism is simplicity itself, because it essentially involves only two master regulatory gene products: one, the plasma membrane antigen and the other, the nuclear-cytosol steroid-receptor protein. More flexible sex-determining mechanisms that operate in fish and amphibians appear infinitely more complicated, perhaps because they have yet to acquire master regulatory genes.

The H-Y antigen, which is the determiner of primary (gonadal) sex in mammals, has been shown to be conserved to the extreme throughout vertebrate evolution. Thus, it has been found in the heterogametic sex of avian as well as amphibian species (WACHTEL et al., 1975a). However, since amphibian sex can readily be reversed by the steroid hormone treatment of larvae, their H-Y antigen appears to be under the control of at least two steroid hormone-receptor proteins, instead of being the master regulatory gene product. Inasmuch as I had rather thoroughly discussed these flexible sex-determining mechanisms of fish and amphibians in my previous book (OHNO, 1967) and since the H-Y antigen does not appear to play the role of the master regulatory gene product in these lower vertebrates, I shall restrain from discussing them in this book. Although H-Y antigen has been identified in the heterogametic female sex of birds, the situation found in the class *Aves* is not as clearly all-or-none as we find it to be in mammals, for male birds too appear to express H-Y antigen, although at a much lower level. Furthermore, the early surgical removal of a functional left ovary of the bird often causes complete sex reversal by testicular development of the right residual gonad. It follows, then, that the H-Y antigen of birds, although ovary-organizing, is flexibly controlled by a gene product of a higher order. Thus I shall not touch upon the sex-determining mechanism of birds in this book either. The point is, that thanks to the presence of master regulatory genes, we have come to understand the mammalian sex-determining mechanism much more clearly than either that which operates in lower vertebrates or that which operates in insects, including the vaunted Drosophila melanogaster.

Chapter 5

The Mammalian Sex Chromosomes

Twenty-five years is the reasonable estimate of our own species' generation time. It follows then that since the birth of Jesus Christ, man has gone through about 80 generations. Any practicing geneticist knows that a period covered by 80 generations is just too short a period for a large population to undergo any sort of striking genetic changes. Meanwhile, populations of viruses, bacteria, and even small rodents must have undergone considerable adaptive changes, for they have gone through many times greater numbers of generations. This observation, illustrates the problem of evolutionary slow-down faced by all large mammalian species. The practice of polygynous matings adapted by many of these species can be viewed as a reasonable attempt at compensation. The polygynous mating system exploits the one-to-one sex ratio that invariably produces a large surplus of adult males. That being the case, each adult male's aggression should be channeled strictly toward other adult males of the same species. In order to do so, adult males should wear tell-tale biological symbols of masculine supremacy so that they cannot be confused with adult females and juveniles of both sexes: hence the development of extreme sexual dimorphism, as already noted. Yet, those heritable traits that made certain males victorious in male-to-male combat must have necessarily benefited females as well as males of the next generation. Accordingly, it is essential to keep a genetic difference between the sexes to the necessary minimum. Once again, we encounter yet another evolutionary paradox: Extreme sexual dimorphism should be manifested on the basis of a minimal sex difference in the genetic constitution.

There are two alternatives for minimizing a genetic difference between males and females. The first alternative is to maintain the X and the Y of the male heterogamety, as well as the Z and the W of the female heterogamety, essentially as two members of a homologous pair, while assigning the sex-determining role to pairs of alleles at a few gene loci. This first alternative has been adapted by a great majority of gonochoristic fish, amphibians, and reptiles, although each class contains a small proportion of exceptional species that are already endowed with the heteromorphic sex chromosome pair (OHNO, 1967, 1974). The advantage of the first alternative lies in the fact that irreversible genetic commitments can be avoided. Indeed, within the same genus of fish, one often sees gonochoristic species coexisting with hermaphroditic species (true synchronous hermaphrodism as well as asynchronous hermaphrodism of both protogynous and protoandrous types). Furthermore, the genetic sex based on the first alternative can readily be reversed by the larval exposure to sex steroids. In the male heterogamety, androgen treatment produces fertile XX males, whereas estrogen treatment causes the development of equally fertile XY females. Nevertheless, one should never be misled into believing that such steroid hormone treatments alter the sex-determining capacity of sex chromosomes. By mating ordinary XY males to sex-reversed XY females, one does obtain YY males; if such YY males are mated to ordinary XX females, in the absence of hormonal manipulations, an all male progeny results, every one of them having the XY sex chromosome constitution (YAMAMOTO, 1961).

Mammals spend their embryonic and fetal life in the maternal environment dominated by female steroid hormones. The above alternative is clearly incompatible with the sexual destiny that has to be shaped during the *in utero* development of individuals. Understandably, mammals have chosen the second alternative and permitted the extensive genetic degeneration of the male-specific Y chromosome, until a few gene loci directly concerned with the primary (gonadal) sex determination are left on it. The heterogametic sex-specific chromosome, which is essentially a genetic dummy containing but a few genes, causes only a minimal sexual difference in the genetic constitution.

In 1959, it was shown that X0 mice are fertile females (WELSHONS and RUSSELL, 1959), whereas the XXY sex chromosome constitution was found in sterile men with the Klinefelter syndrome (JACOBS and STRONG, 1959). Accordingly, it was felt that the mammalian Y chromosome is the male-determining chromosome; therefore, it is no dummy. In this manner, the Y chromosome received a grossly overrated acclaim. The fact is that the Y chromosome knows only one task-which is to divert the embryonic indifferent gonad's inherent tendency to develop toward an ovary and to force it to organize a testis instead. For a task so limited in scope obviously only one or two genes suffice.

Befitting its extremely limited role, the Y chromosome of a vast majority of mammalian species is a rather minute element. Yet, the size is relative, and even the small Y chromosome of man (Fig. 3) contains at least 4 or 5 x 10^7 DNA base pairs that represent nearly ten times the E. coli genome size. Even the minute size of the human Y is in great excess of the very limited task assigned to it. This excess is apparently represented by highly repetitious DNA sequences, many of them Y-chromosome specific, of dubious significance (COOKE, 1976).

Accordingly, most of the long arm of the acrocentric human Y chromosome appears to be readily dispensable. A very tiny fragment of the Y, barely visible under the light microscope and representing only its pericentric region, has apparently been carrying out its assigned task of testicular organization throughout a number of generations in certain human families (the finding of H.P. KLINGER quoted by FRACCARO and LINDSTEN, 1964). As noted in the previous chapter, the DNA sequence of dubious functional significance, not embodying genetic messages, can be added to the genome with no apparent ill effect. In this way, the Y chromosome of exceptional mammalian species, found mostly among rodents, has acquired considerable size without altering its genetic function (Fig. 4).

The mammalian X chromosome, in contrast, is no dummy and the number of gene loci it carries is obviously proportional to its above-average size. In 1964, it was proposed that the original X chromosome of a common mammalian ancestor of some 100 million years ago, comprising roughly 5% of the genome, has been conserved *in toto* by all the divergent mammalian species of today. Consequently, any and all X-linked genes of man should automatically be X-linked in all other mammalian species (OHNO et al., 1964). As shown in Table 1, this proposal by

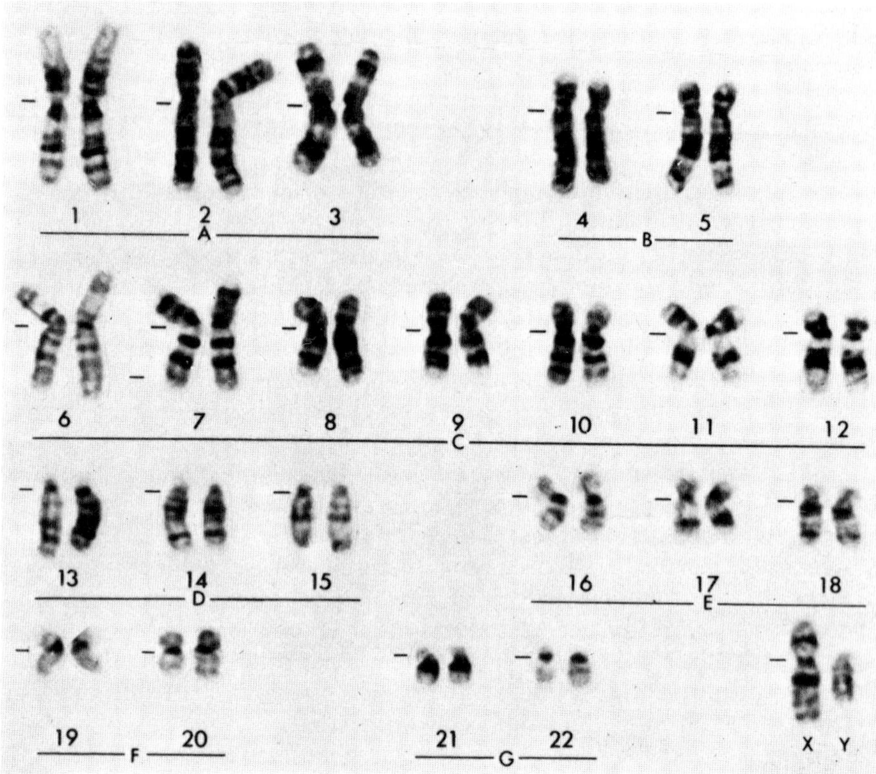

Fig. 3. The G-banded human male karyotype ($2n = 46$). The X of man is the original type comprising roughly 5% of the genome. Within higher primates, even the banding pattern of the X appears to have been conserved. The bulk of the long arm of the Y is made of dispensable constitutive heterochromatin that consists of highly repetitious DNA sequences; some are Y-specific others not. When the Q-banding technique is applied, this portion of the long arm fluoresces brightly (PEARSON et al., 1970) A gift of Dr. C.C. Lin. Univ. of Calgary, Alberta, Canada. Lenses used: 95 x 10

now has become one of the evolutionary laws (MC KUSICK and RUDDLE, 1977). It should be noted that all but two of the X-linked genes listed in Table 1 have nothing whatsoever to do with the act of sex determination or with sex differentiation.

This observation merely reflects the fact that there has never been any evolutionary need to concentrate structural genes for sexual development, such as those specifying sex steroid-synthesizing enzymes, on the X chromosome. To be the X, having a few master regulatory genes for the act of sex determination and differentiation sufficed. The two such genes are listed in Table 1. The X-linkage of the testicular feminization (Tfm) locus has long been suspected in man, but the actual proof of its X-linkage was first obtained in the mouse (LYON and HAWKES, 1970) and subsequently confirmed in man (MEYER et al., 1975). Either by controlling or specifying a single species of the nuclear-cytosol androgen-receptor protein, this locus governs the androgen responsiveness of all types of target cells of the mammalian body (OHNO, 1977a). This then is the master regulatory locus of secondary sex development. Much more shall be said of this locus in Part III.

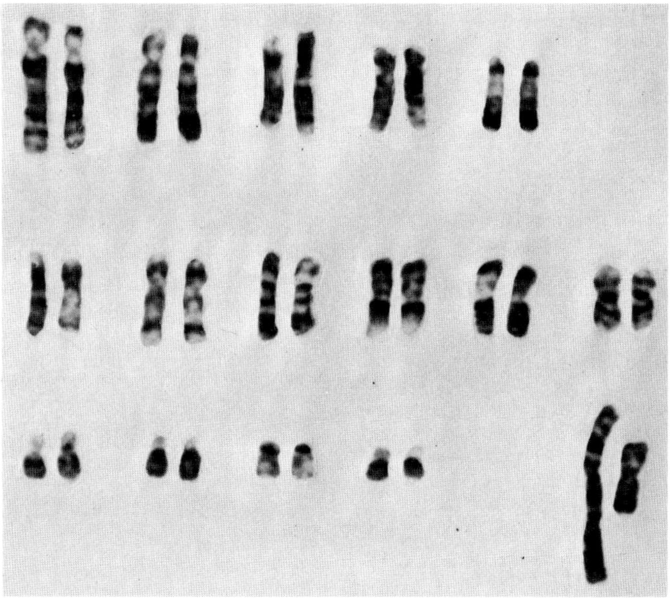

Fig. 4. The G-banded XY karyotype of the wood lemming, *Myopus schisticolor*, $2n = 32$. The X of this species is the duplicate-type, comprising roughly 10% of the genome. However, about half of the long arm of this submediocentric X is comprised of function ally insignificant constitutive heterochromatin, and so is most of the Y which has become quite large due to the accumulation of additional constitutive heterochromatin. This remarkable species is extensively discussed in Chap. 7. A gift of Prof. Alfred Gropp, Lübeck, Germany. Lenses used: 95 x 10

The locus tentatively identified as XY female locus was first identified on the wood lemming, Myopus schisticolor, the karyotype of which is shown in Fig. 4 (FREDGA et al., 1976). Identification of the corresponding locus on the human X, however, has to be implied by rather involved arguments. Here I shall only mention the maternally transmitted familial form of XY women with dysgenetic gonads (STERNBERG et al., 1968), and postpone the involved arguments until Chap. 7. This locus, in cooperation with the Y-linked gene, controls the expression of testis-organizing H-Y antigen. This X-linked locus obviously belongs to the top of the heirarchy of the regulatory system that determines, the primary (gonadal) sex.

While a great majority of mammalian species including man maintain the X chromosome in its original size (see Fig. 3), X chromosomes of exceptional species, again mostly found among rodents, have become considerably larger by the progressive accumulation of functionally trivial DNA material that is known among cytologists as constitutive heterochromatin (Fig. 4). It is a curious fact that the extraordinarily large X chromosome is usually accompanied by the proportionally large Y chromosome. The wood lemming is a good example of this (Fig. 4). Perhaps too great a disparity in their sizes hinders the orderly segregation of the X from the Y during male meiosis. At any rate, the trend toward the accumulation of constitutive heterochromatin, once started, tends to affect the X and the Y together.

Table 1. Evolutionary conservation of mammalian X chromosomes reflected in the homology of X-linked genes

Human X-linked gene product or disease	X-linked in other mammals
Those with functions unrelated to sex	
Glucose-6-phosphate dehydrogenase (of pentose phosphate shunt)	Chimpanzee, horse, donkey, hare, hamster, mouse, kangaroo
Phosphoglycerate kinase (of glycolisis)	Chimpanzee, horse, hamster, mouse, kangaroo
Hypoxanthine-guanine phosphoribosyl transferase (for purine re-utilization)	Chimpanzee, horse, hamster, mouse
Antihemophilic factor VIII (for blood coagulation)	Dog
Antihemophilic factor IX (for blood coagulation)	Dog
X_g erythrocyte antigen	Gibbon
Copper transport deficiency (Menkes kinky-hair syndrome)	Mouse (Brindled alleles)
Vitamin D resistant hypophosphataemic rickets	Mouse
Bruton-type agammaglobulinemia (T-cell dependent B-cell antibody production defect)	Mouse
Anhidrotic ectodermal dysplasia	Cattle
Master sex determining genes for primary and secondary sex	
Testicular feminization: Tfm (nuclear-cytosol androgen-receptor protein defect)	Mouse
XY-female (suppression of testis-organizing H-Y antigen)	Wood lemming

Provided that a breakpoint occurs very near to one or the other terminal end of the X, X-autosome translocations are quite compatible with successful speciation. When earlier cytologists encountered such an X-autosome translocation as a species characteristic, they mistook an intact autosomal homolog of the one which has been united with the X as the second Y chromosome. Even today, a species that has this characteristic type of translocation is said to have the XX/XY_1Y_2 scheme of sex-determining mechanism. The fact is that such a translocation has not altered the sex-determining mechanism in the slightest, for the X here in reality is (X + A), whereas Y_1 is the orginal Y and Y_2 is nothing but A (Fig. 5).

Among the mammalian species that carry this type of translocation, the most notable is the Indian muntjak deer (Muntjacus muntjak) which has the lowest

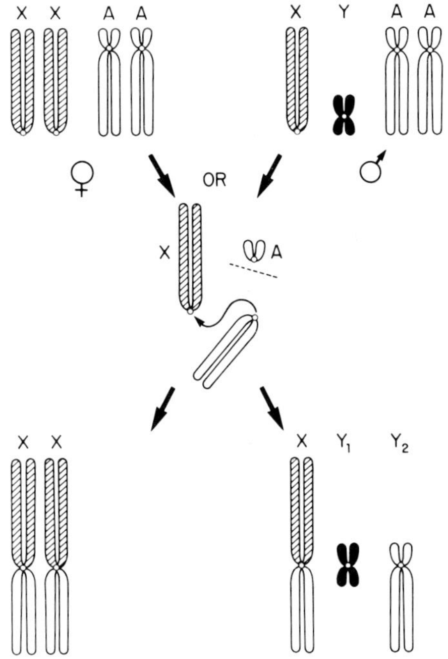

Fig. 5. A change from an ordinary XX/XY system (*top*) to the so-called XX/XY_1Y_2 system (*bottom*) by a simple terminal fusion between the original X and an autosome (*middle*). The original X is hatched, the Y is drawn solid black, an original pair of autosomes is drawn in outline. A slight modification of a figure by FREDGA (1970)

known diploid chromosome number of all mammals; $2n = 7$ for males, $2n = 6$ for females (WURSTER and BENIRSCHKE, 1970). In sharp contrast, its closest living relative, the Chinese muntjak deer (Muntjacus reevesi), maintains the diploid chromosome number of 46 so commonly found among the deer (HSU and BENIRSCHKE, 1968). This pair of species constitutes an extreme example of very extensive chromosomal rearrangements having little effect upon evolutionary diversification. At the other extreme, one sees extensive adaptive radiation having been accomplished with little or no change in the karyotype among whales. Muticetes (baleen whales) and odontocetes (toothed whales) constitute two separate orders that have diverged from each other during Eocene times at the latest, some 50 million years ago. Yet their karyotypes ($2n = 44$) are not readly distinguishable from each other even by modern banding techniques (ARNASSON, 1972).

Terminal Y-autosome fusions (translocations) are also compatible with successful speciation. In this case, an intact autosomal homolog of the chromosome that had fused with the Y has traditionally been mistaken for the second X. Thus, the species involved is said to have the $X_1X_1X_2X_2/X_1X_2Y$ scheme of sex–determining mechanism (Fig. 6). In reality, the X_1 is the true X, whereas X_2 is nothing but A, and Y is (Y + A). Because a functionally critical part of the Y can be submicroscopic, a distinction between (Y + A) and A cannot always be made. Accordingly, the male chromosome constitution of X_1X_2Y can give the appearance of being XO. During male meiosis, however, the X (X_1) unfailingly pairs with one

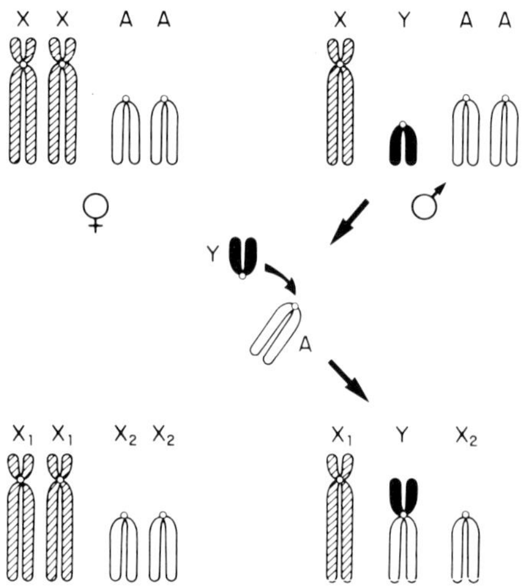

Fig. 6. A change from an ordinary XX/XY system (*top*) to the so-called $X_1X_1X_2X_2/X_1X_2Y$ system (*bottom*) by a simple terminal fusion between the original Y and an autosome (*middle*). The original X, Y, and a pair of autosomes are marked in the same way as Figure 5. A slight modification of a figure by FREDGA (1970)

member of a particular autosomal bivalent, which is (Y+A). The foregoing type of apparent but not real XO males has been identified in a number of Asiatic species of mongooses belonging to the genus *Herpestes* (FREDGA, 1970).

Following the observation that one of the two X chromosomes of female somatic cells remains totally condensed to form the Barr sex chromatin body in interphase nuclei (OHNO et al., 1959), the X–inactivation hypothesis was invented (LYON, 1961; BEUTLER et al., 1962), and this hypothesis has since been confirmed. By this means, even a sexual disparity in the number of X–chromosomes has effectively been minimized.

As far as mammals are concerned, a genetic difference between males and females is indeed kept at the necessary minimum, represented by a few, very possibly one, testis–determining genes residing on the Y chromosome. Furthermore, the identical chromosomal sex–determining mechanism has been conserved by all the divergent mammalian species. Apparent changes of sex chromosomes that sporadically affected a minority of species are not real.

Chapter 6

Initial Gonadal Differentiation and the History of H–Y Antigen

The classical reaggregation experiment done by MOSCONA (1957) not only confirmed the long–held suspicion that the essential information for organogenesis resides on the plasma membrane of component cells, but also revealed that such organogenesis–directing plasma membrane components have been conserved in evolution to the extreme, so that the chick and mouse cells can get together to form one organ. It thus becomes a reasonable assumption that the mammalian Y chromosome directs testicular organization by specifying a male–specific plasma membrane component or components that have been conserved in evolution. Before we proceed any further, however, an outstanding peculiarity of testicular organogenesis should be noted.

Each of the embryonic primordia, as a rule, has but one destiny. For example, of the two diverticula that branch out from the primitive gut, one is destined to be liver, and the other to be pancreas. In contrast, the embryonic indifferent gonad has two developmental alternatives, either to be an ovary or a testis. Furthermore, the basic mammalian embryonic plan is feminine, instead of being neuter in every aspect, and the gonadal development is no exception. Testicular organogenesis should thus be viewed as a superimposed diversion that alters the basic embryonic plan. How soon in the embryonic development of males does such a diversion begin?

a) Initial Gonadal Differentiation

Witschi's original observation (WITSCHI, 1948) that primordial germ cells of mammals do not arise *in situ* in the gonad but instead are first found in the upper yolk sac endoderm above the allantoic rudiment has now become an accepted fact. The initial separation of the germ from the soma, however, is likely to take place considerably earlier, before the yolk sac formation. The migration route of primordial germ cells from the yolk sac to a pair of primitive gonadal ridges on the surface of the mesonephros, first takes them through the splanchnic mesoderm and then through the newly formed mesentery. After making the turn along the coelomic angle, they reach the gonadal ridge (Fig. 7). During migration, some of the mammalian primordial germ cells appear to wander into the blood stream (OHNO and GROPP, 1965). It is of interest to note that this blood–borne route is favored by avian primordial germ cells.

The fate of an emerging gonad appears to be determined by the type of interaction between migrant germ cells and resident somatic cells of the gonadal blastema that is formed at the base of the paired gonadal ridges. Immediately after

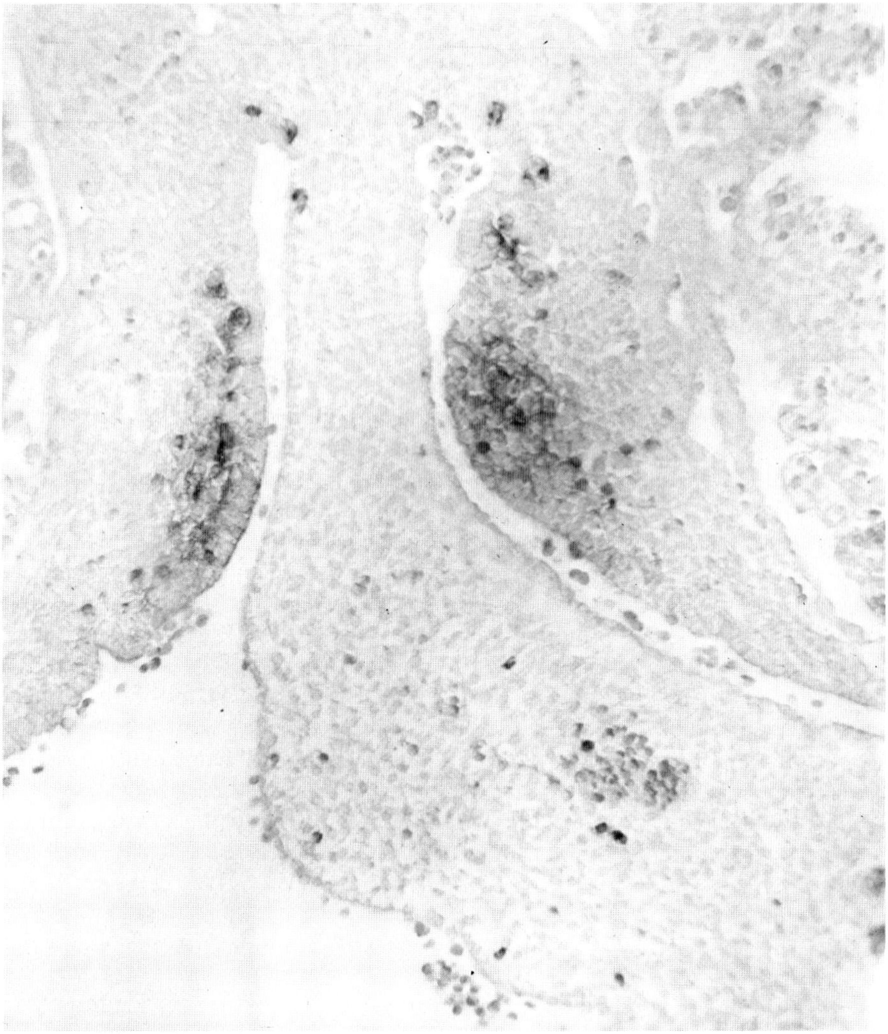

Fig. 7. A transverse section of a cattle embryo (one of the triplets, XX/XY chimaeras) at about the 30th day of the 285-day gestation period; CR length: 12 mm. Because this slide was stained for alkaline phosphatase, positively marked primordial germ cells on their migration route are readily recognizable: about 20 in the dorsal mesentery, 5 at one or the other coelomic angle, and several are seen already in a pair of bulging gonadal ridges. Lenses used: 2.5 x 6

the completion of germ cell migration, it can be debated whether or not the emerging gonad goes through the so-called indifferent or uncommitted state. In cattle, the sex chromosome constitution of very early embryos can readily be determined by cytologic means. In addition, alkaline phosphatase staining distinguishes not only primordial germ cells but also the somatic gonadal blastema. This fortunate combination of favorable conditions enabled us to identify the first sign of sexual differentiation on the fetal cattle gonad. The first sign revealed itself as a sexual difference in the manner of distribution of migrant germ cells. In the XY embryos, germ cells preferentially migrated into the depths and a majority of them soon became lost in the midst of somatic gonadal blastema, whereas those of XX embryos mostly distributed themselves along the gonadal surface and remained there, thus delaying the initial contact between migrant germ cells and resident somatic cells of the gonadal blastema (GROPP and OHNO, 1966). Thus, it would appear that as far as cattle are concerned, the embryonic gonad does not go through an indifferent or uncommitted state. Shortly after the completion of germ cell migration, universally acceptable signs of testicular differentiation are seen in male gonads of every mammalian species studied including man. Testicular cords and rete cords are already recognizable in male gonads of human embryos on the 43rd to the 49th day of the gestational period, which is roughly 280 days (JIRASEK, 1977), in those of mouse embryos at the 15th day of a 20-day-long gestation (PETERS, 1970), and of pig embryos on the 26th day of a gestation period of 115 days (PELLINIEMI, 1975).

The two cell types primarily responsible for testicular tubule formation appear to be precursors of Sertoli cells and underlying mesenchymal cells that furnish the tubular basement membrane. Inasmuch as rete cords successfully develop tubular structures (future collecting tubules) without incorporating primordial germ cells, the role that germ cells play in the tubular formation is questionable. The stuffing of testicular cords with primordial germ cells, on the other hand, is clearly essential to the formation of seminiferous tubules by causing the differentiation of precursor tubular wall cells into Sertoli cells.

My belief is that testicular Sertoli cells and ovarian follicular (granulosa) cells represent two alternate fates of the common precursor cell type, and in this manner, this precursor cell type plays the pivotal role in deciding the fate of an emerging gonad itself. While this precursor cell type in embryonic testes quickly differentiates into recognizable Sertoli cells, e.g., by the 50th day of the 285-day gestation period in cattle, the same cell type in female gonads has to remain as such for a long period before it can manifest its destiny to become follicular (granulosa) cells. First, XX primordial germ cells differentiate into oogonia, and after going through a required number of mitoses, those gonial cells proceed to become oocytes and then go through the first meiotic prophase. Only when individual oocytes suspend their meiosis at the diplotene stage, can the precursor cell type differentiate into follicular cells and organize primordial ovarian follicles by enveloping each dictyate oocyte. In bovine fetal ovaries, the recognizable number of primordial follicles is seen for the first time at about the 120th day of gestation (GROPP and OHNO, 1966).

As far as mammals are concerned, the reason for the much earlier differentiation of male gonads is obvious. Mammalian embryos, males and females alike, grow in the maternal environment dominated by female hormones. This necessitates that the basic embryonic plan become inherently feminine, for by so doing, not only ovarian differentiation but also feminine extragonadal development is made independent and autonomous, not requiring hormonal induction. There is no reason for fetal mammalian ovaries to acquire endocrine functions. As an inevitable consequence, extragonadal masculine development had to become an androgen–dependent process. Accordingly, as soon as the embryonic gonad develops into a testis, it immediately has to fulfill its role as an endocrine organ. Indeed freshly differentiated testicular Sertoli cells immediately begin to secrete an antimüllerian factor to prevent an autonomous differentiation of müllerian ducts into female genital tracts, fallopian tubules, and uterus (Tran et al., 1977). More importantly, Leydig cells have to begin the synthesis of testosterone, for Wolffian ducts can differentiate into male genital tracts only in the presence of testosterone. In human male fetuses, Leydig cells begin active androgen synthesis as early as the 60th day of gestation, and this activity reaches a peak at the 90th day, when Leydig cells make up more than half the volume of the fetal testis (Pelliniemi and Niemi, 1969). As soon as these fetal assignments have been completed, both Sertoli and Leydig cells become quiescent. However, this does not imply that a diversion of the inherently feminine embryonic plan of the gonad can only take place at the very beginning of an emerging gonad. As we shall later discuss more fully, the testicular transformation of bovine freemartin XX gonads occurs very late, after considerable differentiation of the female gonad as an ovary has already occurred. It would appear that the slow leisurely differentiation process of mammalian ovaries can be diverted toward testicular development not only at the very beginning of gonadal development but also at various times thereafter. A specific plasma membrane component or components responsible for testicular organogenesis must necessarily play a dominant role over the inherently feminine embryonic plan.

b) The History of H-Y Antigen

Traditionally, immunologists have been most adept at identifying various plasma membrane components for, when confronted with viable cells, the host mounts humoral antibody as well as cell-mediated immune response specifically directed against nonself plasma membrane components of the cells with which it is challenged. Indeed, the plasma membrane component responsible for mammalian testicular organogenesis was first identified as a minor histocompatibility antigen. Twenty-three years ago Eichwald and Silmser (1955) reported the rather unexpected finding that within an inbred strain, females consistently rejected male skin grafts. Since the rejection was obviously caused by a male-specific antigen, it was identified as H-Y. However, it soon became evident that the consistent rejection of male skin grafts by females, with a mean graft survival time of 25.6 days or so, occurs only in certain inbred strains such as C57BLACK/6 (B6) and C57BLACK/10 (B10); as many as 87% of the females of various other strains, such as C3H and CBA, permanently accept male skin grafts. Lively debates ensued as to whether only males of certain inbred strains are endowed with H-Y antigen. The cause of strain differences in rejecting male grafts however, was eventually identified. It was the H-2 haplotypes of the MHC (major histocompatibility) gene complex that determine the manner in which females respond to male grafts. The strong rejector strains such as B6 and B10 are H-2^b, whereas notorious nonrejectors such as C3H and CBA are H-2^k. H-2^a and H-2^d strains such as A and BALB/c represent weak inconsistent rejectors. I shall only mention that congenic strains, such as BALB/c versus BALB.B, differing genetically only at the MHC gene complex (H-2^d versus H-2), served as very important tools and that D.W. Bailey, R.E. Billingham, D.J. Gasser, A. Langerova, W.K. Silvers, S.S. Wachtel, and I.J. Weissman among others contributed prominently to elucidating the dominant role that H-2 haplotypes play in the manner of rejection of H-Y incompatible grafts. Obviously, the influence of H-2 haplotypes is through two independent sources: H-2D and H-2K genes of the male target, as well as Ir (immune response) genes residing within the MHC of female responders. It was thus shown that even H-2^k males of the nonrejector strain are endowed with a healthy dose of H-Y antigen, for H-2^k/H-2^b F1 females vigorously rejected male H-2^k grafts, with a mean graft survival time of only 24.2 days.

These extensive transplantation studies carried out by the above-named investigators soon revealed the distinct uniqueness of the H-Y antigen. Whereas genetic polymorphism is the hallmark of all other histocompatibility gene loci of the mouse, H-Y antigen is obviously monomorphic. An allelism of the H-Y antigen locus, if it exists at all, must represent a very inconsequential genetic difference (HILDEMAN et al., 1970). In hindsight, this apparent monomorphism was a very important clue, for a gene product that has remained so invariant cannot possibly be a mere minor histocompatibility antigen. Nevertheless, in an apparent absence of genetic polymorphism, the postulated Y-linkage of the H-Y structural gene cannot be substantiated. Accordingly, the opinion that the H-Y structural gene might in fact be residing either within or in very close proximity to the MHC gene complex had often been expressed (e.g., STEINMULLER and EICHWALD, 1971). In fact, this uncertainty about the H-Y structural gene location is still a thorn in our understanding of the mammalian primary (gonadal) sex-determining mechanism. We shall discuss this problem further in the last chapter of Part II.

A genetic difference at the MHC gene complex causes very violent graft rejections that completely mask whatever other genetic differences might have existed at one or more of the minor histocompatibility gene loci. Furthermore, as far as graft rejections are concerned, H-Y is but one of many minor histocompatibility antigens. It follows then that demonstration by graftings of the H-Y antigen is possible only in those laboratory species in which inbred strains are readily available. Understandably, the next mammalian species in which the male-specific occurence of the H-Y antigen was demonstrated was the laboratory rat (BILLINGHAM and SILVERS, 1959). In this species too, MHC dependence of the H-Y incompatible graft rejection mechanism was noted. The ZW/ZZ scheme of chromosomal sex-determing mechanisms based on the female heterogamety operates in the class Aves. When inbred strains of the chicken became available it was soon shown that, in birds, it is the homogametic male sex that rejects isologous female grafts. This avian female-specific histocompatibility antigen might as well have been called H-W antigen (GILMORE, 1967). By using fin grafts, the heterogametic sex-specific histocompatibility antigen has also been demonstrated in a teleost fish, Platypoecilus maculatus (KALLMAN 1970). In this tiny fish species, the XX/XY male heterogamety and the ZW/ZZ female heterogamety operate side by side in different populations. While the findings noted above indicate the universal occurence in vertebrates of a heterogametic sex-specific plasma membrane antigen, as long as graft rejections remained the only means of demonstrating its presence, the evolutionary raison d'etre of the H-Y or H-W antigen had to remain an enigma. Even today, this is still true of all other minor histocompatibility antigens.

The first attempts at developing a serologic assay method for the H-Y antigen were apparently made by HAUSCHKA et al. (1959). However, we owe development of workable serologic methods to various individuals who have been, at one time or another associated with the laboratory of E.A. Boyse.

In our laboratory, we routinely raise humoral H-Y antibody in B6 (H-2^b) females by five weekly injections of 25 to 5 x 10^6 each of isologous male spleen and lymphode cells. It is important to use the cell type that is shared in common by males and females alike as the source of the H-Y antigen. When confronted with male lymphoid cells, the isologous female immune system would recognize the H-Y antigen as the one and only nonself component on the male cell plasma membrane. However, if confronted with a male-specific cell type such as spermatozoa or testicular Leydig cells, even the isologous female immune system would now recognize as nonself not only H-Y but also many other cell type-specific differentiation antigens on the male plasma membrane, thus generating a multitude of antimale antibodies in addition to the H-Y antibody. However, even the use of male lymphoid cells as the H-Y antigen source does not automatically insure the production of uncontaminated H-Y antibody. Often, the tolerance of H-Y antigen appears to be induced on immunized females by weekly injections. Such females never yield H-Y antibody. Conversely, we often find H-Y antibody to be contaminated with other cytotoxic antibody directed against male and female epidermal cells of BALB/c. Since male BALB epidermal cells are the target cell type of our choice in the cytotoxicity test of H-Y antibody, such contaminating antibody or antibodies have to be removed by exhaustive absorption using female BALB epidermal cells. The generally feeble immune response that female mice mount against H-Y antigen, while a nuisance to investigators, is readily understandable. As pregnant females are invariably exposed to H-Y antigen disseminated by male fetuses *in utero*, natural selection must have made certain that females do not mount too effective an immune response against so important an antigen as the testis-organizing H-Y. Indeed, we find H-Y antibody to be almost always of the IgM class. This certainly suggests the presence, in females, of suppressor T cells that prevent H-Y antibody-producing clones from making switch from IgM to IgG. A point of interest here is the observation that H-Y antibody can be raised in nonrejector (H-2^k) and strong rejector (H-2^b) strains alike (GOLDBERG et al., 1972).

Despite sporadic claims to the contrary, we have never been able to demonstrate the cytotoxic effect of H-Y antibody on male spleen and other hematopoietic cells. The three well-verified cytotoxic target cell types of H-Y antibody are: (1) epididymal spermatozoa (GOLDBERG et al., 1971); (2) male epidermal cells obtained from the tail by the double trypsin treatment-after the first strong treatment, thick dermis is peeled off from a thin layer of epidermis. Then clumps of epidermal cells are obtained by scraping the inner surface of epidermis. These clumps are dispersed by a second mild treatment to yield a free cell suspension (SCHEID et al., 1972). (3) Preimplantation male embryos of the 8-cell stage from which *zona pelucida* have been removed by pronase treatment (KRCO and GOLDBERG, 1976).

The first obstacle encountered in performing the H-Y antibody cytotoxicity test, using any of the preceding three target cell types is the almost invariably present nonspecific cytotoxicity shown by liquid nitrogen-stored rabbit or guinea pig sera used as the source of complement. We routinely screen a large number of agarose-absorbed guinea pig complements and choose only those that show no appreciable cytotoxicity to male BALB thymus cells. By this screening, we have been able to keep the complement control killing value to about 30% (Fig. 8). Since few investigators, excluding myself, are capable of distinguishing under the microscope live spermatozoa from trypan blue-stained dead spermatozoa, the target cell type of choice in this laboratory became male BALB epidermal cells. An additional advantage of this cell type is the availability of female counter parts. The maximal killing by H-Y antibody seldom exceeds 60% of the male epidermal cells and a good H-Y antibody maintains this cytotoxic strength until 1:16 dilution; the real dilution in a reaction mixture is 1:48 = 1:16 x 1:3. The cytotoxicity is absolutely male specific (Fig. 8). Male preimplantation embryos of the 8-cell stage appear extraordinarily sensitive to the cytotoxic effect of H-Y antibody. When we have karyotyped surviving embryos that endured the H-Y antibody treatment on a few occasions, we encountered nothing but the XX chromosome constitution among them, thus suggesting 100% lysis of male embryos. These 8-cell stage embryos, however, are too expensive a cell type for daily use as the cytotoxic target of H-Y antibody.

The reason that we use male epidermal cells of BALB/c strain is that the cytotoxic sensitivity to H-Y antibody of male target cells is greatly influenced by their H-2 haplotypes (SCHEID et al., 1972). Those of $H\text{-}2^b$ and $H\text{-}2^d$ strains are most sensitive, whereas male $H\text{-}2_k$ cells are most resistant and male $H\text{-}2^a$ cells occupy the intermediate postion (Fig. 9).Thus, one should never use male $H\text{-}2^k$ cells, such as those of C3H and CBA strains, for the H-Y antibody cytotoxicity test. Cu-

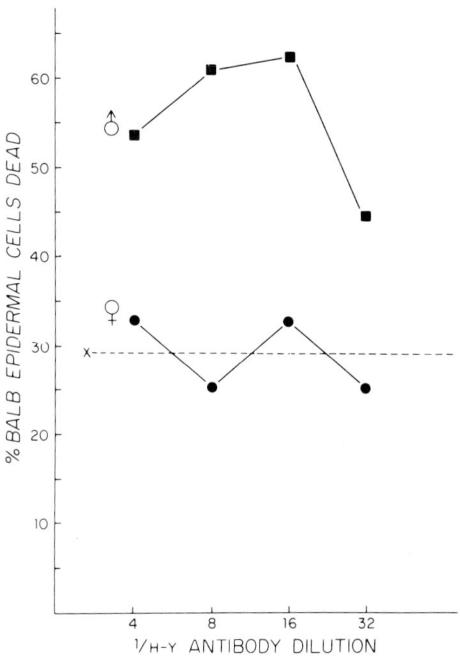

Fig. 8. The male-specific cytotoxicity of good, uncontaminated H-Y antibody on male and female BALB epidermal cells. Agarose-absorbed guinea pig complements were used. The complement control killing was 29%

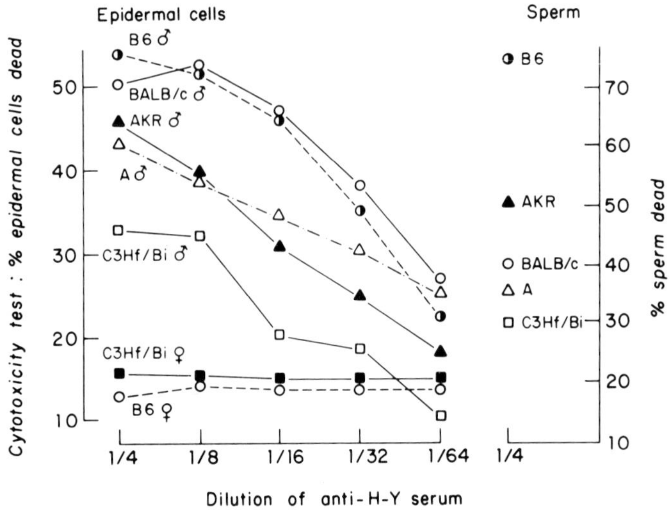

Fig. 9. The influence of H-2 haplotypes on the cytotoxic sensitivity to H-Y antibody of male epidermal cells and spermatozoa. The most susceptible B6 and BALB are H-2^b and H-2^d, while A and AKR, being of H-2^a strains, are intermediate in their sensitivities. The very resistant C3H is H-2^k. This figure was slightly modified from Fig. 4 of SCHEID, et al (1972)

riously, the same holds true for male 8-cell stage embryos, despite the generally accepted belief that H-2 antigens are not expressed so early in embryonic development. Although male B6 or B10 epidermal cells, being H-2^b, are as sensitive to H-Y antibody as male BALB cells (Fig. 9), melanin granules present in a considerable proportion of the former interferes with the trypan blue dye exclusion test. BALB, being albino, lacks melanin granules.

Establishment of the above-noted H-Y antigen assay systems opened an entirely new era of the study of H-Y antigen, for the presence or absence of H-Y antigen can now be studied on cells of any other species by the antibody absorption test. Here it should be emphasized that H-Y antigen levels, even of mouse cells, should be quantitatively assessed by the antibody absorption test and never by the direct cytotoxicity test, for the simple reason that cytotoxic sensitivity to H-Y antibody does not reflect the number of H-Y antigen sites on the target cell plasma membrane. I have already noted H-2 dependent cytotoxic sensitivities of male target cells to H-Y antibody (Fig. 9). Yet H-2 haplotypes do not influence the number of H-Y antigen sites per male target cell, because the H-Y antibody absorption test reveals that male epidermal cells of the resistant C3H (H-2^k and sensitive BALB (H-2^d) strains are endowed with an equal number of H-Y antigen sites. Reflecting the crucial role that H-Y antigen plays in their differentiation, fetal and newborn testicular cells (primordial germ cells less than Sertoli and Leydig cells) absorb as much H-Y antibody as adult male epidermal cells, yet these testicular cells are totally resistant to the cytotoxic effect of H-Y antibody.

We customarily determine the number of H-Y antigen sites per cell by the following absorption procedure: (1) The strength of 50 μl of anti-H-Y serum (usually diluted 1/4) is adjusted so that 2 x 10^6 adult male BALB spleen cells absorb out exactly 50% of its male-specific cytotoxicity. (2) Each H-Y antiserum of the above strength is then absorbed with a certain number of test cells to form a graduated series: 2, 4, 8, 16 ...... × 10^6 cells (the absorption is always carried out on ice for 45 min; the residual cytotoxicity of absorbed H-Y antibody is titrated on male BALB epidermal cells again in the presence of agarose-absorbed guinea pig complements); (3) in this manner, the number of test cells required for 50% absorption of the H-Y antibody's male-specific cytotoxicity is determined (Fig. 10); (4) the above determination is tested by doubling the determined number (this doubled number should represent the minimal number of test cells required for 100% absorption. Needless to say, the cell number required for 50% H-Y antibody absorption is inversely proportional to the number of H-Y antigen sites per cell).

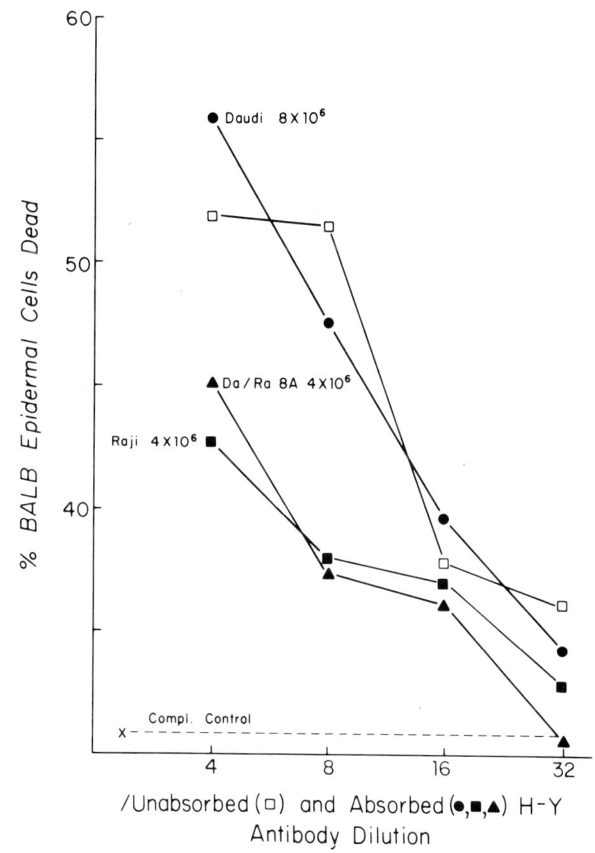

Fig. 10. A good example of H-Y antibody absorption tests performed on two male human pseudodiploid Burkitt lymphoma lines, Raji and Daudi, as well as on Daudi x Raji 8A, a somatic hybrid between the two. 4 x 10^6 Raji cells, as well as the same number of Daudi x Raji 8A cells, achieved 50% absorption of the male-specific cytotoxicity. In sharp contrast, even 8 x 10^6 Daudi cells have yet to show their H-Y antibody absorption capacity. As many as 22 x 10^6 Daudi cells are required for 50% absorption. This peculiarity of Daudi is discussed in detail in Chap. 8, Sect. c

When an extensive series of such H-Y antibody absorption tests was performed by WACHTEL et al., (1975a), the extreme evolutionary conservation of H-Y antigen throughout adaptive radiations of vertebrates was revealed. Male cells of all other mammalian species tested, including man, readily absorbed out the male-specific cytotoxicity of the H-Y antibody, as well as the corresponding cell types of male mice. On the other hand, no cross-reacting materials were found on female cells, even if as many as 40×10^6 cells were used for absorption. In birds, it was now heterogametic female cells that consistently absorbed more H-Y antibody than male cells. In amphibian cells, whichever sex that was heterogametic, absorbed more H-Y antibody. In Rana pipiens (leopard frog), XY male cells absorbed more, whereas in Xenopus laevis (African water frog), female ZW cells absorbed more. The plasma membrane component that remained so invariant throughout vertebrate evolution cannot possibly be a mere minor histocompatibility antigen. It must have been performing the same critical function through all these several hundred million years.

Chapter 7

Testis-Organizing Function of H-Y Antigen

The extreme evolutionary conservatism displayed by H-Y antigen is reminiscent of the similar and even more extreme conservatism displayed by histone IV. The very exact and invariant function must have been assigned to H-Y antigen throughout the age of mammals. As far as mammals are concerned, the role of the H-Y antigent almost had to be that of the primary (gonadal) sex determiner. H-Y antigen must have been diverting the emerging gonad's inherent tendency to develop into an ovary, causing it to organize a testis instead.

There is one apparent drawback to the above assumption. An inevitable corollary to the above is that the same antigen in birds must have been playing the opposite role, that of the ovary organizer. At first glance, such a complete reversal of the role by the same plasma membrane component appeared improbable to say the least. However, it was recalled that there have been a number of inexplicable observations and that these observations suddenly made good sense, if one postulated a complete reversal of the primary (gonadal) sex-determining role by the same gene product between mammals and birds.

For a number of years, J-P. Weniger's group in Strasbourg has been reporting a series of interesting but very puzzling experiments. When mammalian and avian embryonic testis were cultured side by side in very close contact on an agar plate for several days, inexplicable feminization of the avian testis occurred: for example, the chick and bovine embryonic testis combination reported by AKRAM and WENIGER (1968). This phenomenon can now be explained. Upon reaching the avian embryonic testis, the H-Y antigen disseminated by a mammalian testis functions as an ovary-organizing H-Y antigen. In cattle, vascular anastomosis between heterosexual dizygotic twin embryos causes the testis-like development of the female gonad which then secretes testosterone to partially masculinize her own body (freemartin condition). In the chicken and the duck, a similar vascular anastomosis develops between dizygotic twins of a double yolked egg. In the heterosexual combination, it is the testis of a chromosomal male that is affected and becomes ovary-like (LUTZ and LUTZ-OSTERTAG, 1958). In mammals, XY male cells disseminate testis-organizing H-Y antigen, while in birds, ZW female cells disseminate ovary-organizing H-Y antigen. Satisfied with the above considerations, we have proposed the testis-organizing role for mammalian H-Y antigen (WACHTEL et al., 1975 b).

Inasmuch as the fate of gonads is the only concern of the mammalian chromosomal sex-determining mechanism, the above proposal predicts that in a very strict sense the mammalian primary (gonadal) sex should be determined not so much by the presence or absence of the Y chromosome but by the expression or nonexpression of the H-Y antigen. Thus, we began to look for exceptional species and individuals upon which the above proposal could be tested.

a) Normal XO Males of the Mole Vole, *Ellobius lutescens,* and Fertile XY or Even XYY Females of the Wood Lemming, *Myopus schisticolor*

As far as the chromosomal sex-determining mechanism is concerned, most venturesome species are found in the rodent family, Microtinae. Thus, OY males and XO females were first reported in the creeping vole, Microtus oregoni (MATTHEY, 1958). Subsequently, however, both sexes of this species were shown to be gonosomic mosaics: $2n = 17/18$ (OY/XY) for the male, $2n = 18/17$ (XX/XO) for the female. As usual, XY zygotes gave rise to males, but the X was preferentially eliminated from the male germ line, so that all the females started from XO zygotes. Nevertheless, a hazard of involving two heterogametic germ lines in the mating was avoided by the restitution of two Xs to oogonia (OHNO et al., 1966). The last known enigma is the mole vole, Ellobius lutescens: $2n = 17$. The apparent XO chromosome constitution has been confirmed on both the germ and the soma of both sexes (MATTHEY, 1964; CASTRO-SIERRA and WOLF, 1968). As noted before, "apparent" XO males of mongoose species belonging to the genus Herpestes are in truth XY. During male meiosis, the pairing between the X and the Y-carrying autosome insures the orderly segregation of the X from the Y (FREDGA, 1970). The XO males of the mole vole, on the other hand, appear to be genuine: There is no specific autosome segregating from the X at the end of the first meiotic division (CASTRO-SIERRA and WOLF, 1968). Accordingly, the mating of this species obviously involves two heterogametic germ lines that should cause 50 % loss of the zygotes. Indeed, when pregnant females of the mole vole and the creeping vole were examined, at least 50% preimplantation loss of the zygotes was evident in the former, whereas no sign of excessive zygotic loss was seen in the latter, as expected (LYAPNOVA et al., 1975). Although the sex-determining role was suggested to be a polymorphism of the largest pair of autosomes (DE LA MAZA and SAWYER, 1976), this scheme predicts 75% zygotic loss. Inasmuch as autosomal polymorphism as revealed by modern banding techniques is the rule rather than the exception in noninbred populations, such instant assignment of the sex-determining role to an autosomal polymorphism appears untenable. When the expression of H-Y antigen was studied on the mole vole, XO males were found to express H-Y antigen in the same manner as XY males of any other mammalian species, while no H-Y antigen was detectable in XO females (NAGAI and OHNO, 1977). Thus, in the mole vole, the primary (gonadal) sex is, indeed, determined not by the presence or absence of the Y chromosome, but by the expression or nonexpression of the H-Y antigen.

The 1:1 sex ratio is the inevitable consequence of the XX/XY chromosomal sex-determining mechanism and as it operates in mammals, a large surplus of males is created. The sex ratio of 1:3 or even 1:6 in favor of females appears to be more suitable to meet the reproduktive needs of mammals. Yet, as far as we know, only a very few species have managed to alter the monotonous 1:1 sex ratio to substantially reduce the number of male births. The Scandinavian wood lemming

(Myopus schisticolor) and its distant Alaskan kin, Dicrostonyx torquatus, are those few ingenious species. The mechanism by which wood lemmings achieve this rare feat has been revealed by the study of FREDGA et al. (1976). The karyotype of this species ($2n=32$) has already been shown in Fig. 4. In essence, three types of females exist in this species, and only one type consists of conventional XX females that produce equal numbers of males and females. The second type of female is XX also, but these females produce three times more females than males, and a third of the female offspring are XY. When mated to ordinary XY males, this third type of female, the XY female, produces nothing but females, half of which are again XY. These fertile XY females avoid the hazard of involving two heterogametic germ lines in the mating by utilizing the same device that XO females of the creeping vole use (as discussed on page 40). The Y is eliminated, and then the X is duplicated to give an XX constitution to oogonia in the XY females. An X-linked mutation is clearly responsible for the production of fertile XY females. The second type of XX female is heterozygous for this mutation, whereas the third type of XY female is hemizygotic. Because these XY females transmit nothing but the mutated X to their progeny through homozygous XX oocytes, the production of all female progeny is readily understandable.

More detailed studies by Gropp and his colleagues on the domesticated stock of Fritz Frank revealed that there can even be XYY females. They have also found what Gropp calls Durchbrenner among fertile XY females. These exceptional "escapers" do produce a few XY sons (GROPP et al., 1976). It would appear that the device that restores two Xs to the female germ line of these XY females is not beyond occassional error and that XY oocytes can arise. XY sons of these escaper XY females then are truly paradoxical products in that their Y is of maternal origin, whereas their X is paternally derived.

Needless to say, the wood lemming exposed the proposed testis-organizing function of the H-Y antigen to the severest test imaginable. Because these fertile XY females receive their Ys from obviously fertile fathers, there can be no genetic defect on their Ys, yet an X-linked mutation renders the Ys testis-determining potential totally powerless. According to the proposal, what a mutated X suppresses has to be the expression of the H-Y antigen. While XY males were H-Y antigen positive, no detectable amount of H-Y antigen was found on these fertile XY females (WACHTEL et al., 1976b). The findings on the two exceptioal species, Ellobius lutescens and Myopus schisticolor, indeed reveals that in a strict sense, the primary (gonadal) sex of mammals is determined not so much by the presence or absence of the Y but the expression or nonexpression of the H-Y antigen.

b) Exceptional Individuals among Man and Other Mammalian Species: XX Males and XY Females

Even among the majority of mammalian species in which an ordinary XX/XY system operates, XX and even XO males, as well as XY females, do occur as exceptions. In man, for example, the incidence of XX males is said to be one in several thousand live births (DE LA CHAPELLE, 1972). We shall discuss various heritable forms of XX males first.

In the mouse, an autosomal dominant Sxr gene, transmitted through a carrier XY, Sxr/- father to half of his progeny, produces XX, Sxr/- males (CATTANACH et al., 1971). XX human males, caused by a paternally transmitted dominant gene, have also been reported (KASDAN et al., 1973). In the goat, on the other hand, XX males and XX true hermaphrodites are the homozygotes for an autosomal gene, Polled. As a cause of hornlessness, this gene is dominant; but, as a cause of testicular development in the absence of the Y, the same gene behaves as a recessive (HAMERTON et al., 1969).

As to the apparently nonheritable form of XX human males when the X-linked Xg blood group was informative, a striking peculiarity was noted: i.e., XX males out of Xga+ fathers and Xga− mothers were Xga−. They behaved as though they received both X s from their mothers and none from their fathers. It was suggested that a meiotic exchange between the X and the Y of the father transferred the Xga+ gene from the X to the Y, and the X, in turn, received the testis-determining gene from the Y, hence, testicular development in the absence of the Y (FERGUSON-SMITH, 1966). An alternative explanation offered was that they all started from the XY zygote, but a mitotic nondisjunction first eliminated the Y, then duplicated the maternally derived X to produce the XX cell line, which then became preponderant. According to this view, the persistence of an original XY line in their gonads is responsible for testicular organization (DE LA CHAPELLE, 1972). The occasional identification of XO human males can be taken as evidence that supports the latter alternative (BOTTURA and FERRARI, 1962).

In the absence of mosaicism, can XX males arise that do not receive the testis-determining gene from the Y? The situation found in the pig appears to give an affirmative answer. The condition of intersexuality is extremely common in the pig: Up to 4% of newborn piglets may be affected in some litters, and the frequency of affected litters may be as high as 28%. Here again, the most commonly seen aberration in affected piglets is testicular development in the absence of the Y, yielding XX males or male pseudohermaphrodites. To the extent that the incidence differs in different breeds and lines, there certainly is a genetic component. Nevertheless, within a given breed, this condition does not appear to be a heritable trait, more being found among larger litters. These XX males or pseudohermaphrodites are not XX/XY chimeras as are bovine freemartins. Porcine freemartins have been identified as a separate condition (BREEUWSMA, 1970).

In conformity with the proposed testis-determining function of H-Y antigen, XX, Sxr/- male mice expressed H-Y antigen in the absence of the Y (BENNETT et al., 1977; WACHTEL, et al., 1977). Whether or not an autosomal Sxr gene, in fact, is the Yderived testis-determining gene shall be discussed in the last chapter of Part II. In humans, H-Y antigen studies in four XX males and three XX true hermaphrodites have been reported (WACHTEL et al., 1976a). All of them were found to be H-Y antigen positive. While these findings constituted additional evidence in support of the proposed testis-organizing function of the H-Y antigen, the problem of how was expressed the H-Y antigen in the absence of the Y remained unresolved. It would have been more informative if the paternally inherited form of XX males noted earlier had been included in the above study. One XX male had an extra piece of chromosomal material attached to the short arm tip of one X. This was thought to represent a functionally critical piece of the Y. Among cultured fibroblasts from another XX male, one XXY mitotic figure among many more XX was encountered. Testicular development in this XX male could have been due to the XXY cell line that he harbored in his gonads. The H-Y antigen test, however, was done not on his gonadal cells but on his peripheral blood leukocytes as well as on cultured fibroblasts. The observed H-Y antigen level of these two cell types could not possibly be attributable to XXY cells alone that were a barely recognizable minority. Accordingly, in this particular case, the transfer of H-Y antigen from XXY to XX cells may have to be invoked to explain the result. In our own experience with a few copies of XX human males and XX true hermaphrodites, we too found H-Y antigend expressed in all of these XX patients, although at a subnormal level; 70 – 80%.

In the laboratory mouse, fertile X0 females ovulate XO eggs, thus producing some X0 daughters (WELSHONS and RUSSELL, 1959). On the other hand, both normally XO females of the creeping vole and the fertile XY females of the wood lemming have developed a device for restoring the XX sex chromosome constitution to their oogonia, as already noted. In large mammals with long gestation periods such as man and the horse, XO oocytes undergo fetal or neonatal degeneration. Since XO females of these species are not equipped with a device for restoring XX oogonia, they develop as sterile females with dysgenetic ovaries. I have already mentioned that a maternally transmitted mutation responsible for the heritable form of XY women with pure gonadal dysgenesis (STERNBERG et al., 1968) might be homologous to an X-linked mutation that produces fertile XY wood lemming females. This assumption is valid only if the human XY "ovary" suffers the same dysgenetic fate as the X0 gonad. However, it should be recalled that exceptional XY wood lemming females (Druchbrenner of Gropp) do produce functional XY eggs. Furthermore, when XX/XY chimeric mice produced by blastocyst fusions develop as fertile females, functional XY oocytes have been found in their ovaries (EVANS et al., 1977). Accordingly, the possibility exists that an X-linked mutation of man homologous to that seen in the wood lemming might produce fertile XY women. If such proves to be the case, one has to conclude that an X-linked mutation that produces XY phenotypic females with pure gonadal dysgenesis represents a different mutation, albeit of the same locus.

As already noted, gonadal dysgenesis in man is most often associated with the X0 condition, but the XX form is also known. The XY condition differs from X0 gonadal dysgenesis by the absence of stigmata that comprise the Turner syndrome, and from the XX form by a very high incidence of gonadal tumors. The extensive biopsy and autopsy studies summarized by REHDER (1976) indicated that gonadal tumors that develop in XY women with pure gonadal dysgenesis are almost invariably of the testicular type. As far as the XY phenotypic female is concerned, the primary (gonadal) sex appears to be a form of dysgenetic testis. The development of female somatic sex structure can be attributed to the lack of fetal testosterone production caused by dysgenesis of the H-Y antigen-organized testis. Not surprisingly, each of the several XY women with pure gonadal dysgenesis whom we have studied expressed the H-Y antigen, although at a noticeably subnormal level. Wachtel has had the same experience. Regretfully, neither has studied the maternally transmitted heritable form. All in all, studies on exceptional individuals of man, and other mammalian species too appear to have supported a notion that the mammalian primary sex is determined by the expression or nonexpression of the H-Y antigen and not necessarily by the presence or absence of the Y chromosome.

c) Moscona Experiments: Testicular Cells Lysostripped of H-Y Antigen Organize Ovarian-Follicle-Like Aggregates

The remarkable existence of fertile XY wood lemming females revealed to us that in the absence of H-Y antigen expression, XY gonadal cells readily organize an ovary. Can one repeat the same feat *in vitro* by performing Moscona-type reaggregation experiments? The fact that a serologically detectable H-Y antigen has been conserved in evolution to the extreme (WACHTEL et al., 1975a) indicates that this immunoreactive part probably represents the functionally critical active site of the H-Y antigen. It follows then that by the proper use of H-Y antibody, one should be able to deprive male gonadal cells of their testis-organizing capacity. In the presence of an excess of antibody the plasma membrane antigen complexed with that antibody has been found to gather over one pole of the cell; the "capping" phenomenon (TAYLOR et al., 1971). These capped antigen-antibody complexes are subsequently consumed by lysosomes of the cell, thus its cytoplasm becomes denuded of that particular antigen for a period of several hours, the "lysostripping" phenomenon (CULLEN et al., 1973). Fig. 11 schematically illustrates the capping and subsequent lysostripping process.

As already noted, H-Y antibody at its best is not a very potent antibody. However, perhaps because it is mostly of the IgM class, we found that H-Y antibody alone, without the addition of xenogenic antimouse IgM antibody, can cause the lysostripping of H-Y antigen. Inasmuch as H-Y antibody is cytotoxic in the presence of complements to male mouse epidermal cells but not to fetal and newborn testicular cells, the procedure for lysostripping of H-Y antigen had to be worked out on adult male BALB epidermal cells. When these cells were first incubated with a large excess of H-Y antibody at a 1:5 dilution for 45 min on ice and then for another hour at 37°C, the lysostripping of H-Y antigen was effectively accomplished. When these treated cells, after washing, were subsequently exposed to fresh H-Y antibody and guinea pig complement, they remained totally resistant to the cytotoxic effect of H-Y antibody for a period of 6-8 h. For this period of time, male BALB epidermal cell cytoplasm apparently remained denuded of H-Y antigen.

As described in Chap. 6, the mammalian ovary differentiates at a considerably slower pace than the testis, and it does not acquire its true histologic distinction until primordial follicles are formed. For this reason, we chose newborn rather than fetal BALB testicular cells for our Moscona-type reaggregation experiments. Newborn mouse ovaries are full of primordial follicles, each follicle consisting of a dictyate oocyte surounded by one or more layers of follicular cells. The experimental procedure employed is illustrated schematically in Fig. 12 (see page 46).

In short, free testicular cells lysostripped of H-Y antigen were immediately subjected to the rotation culture for a period of 16 h and their reaggregated structures were compared with those found in the control culture. The difference was remarkable. While the control culture yielded a large number of short but tortuous tubular structures (Fig. 13, left), the H-Y antibody-treated culture yielded numerous spherical aggregates (Fig. 13, right), each of which under close scrutiny was found to consist of a large primordial germ cell surrounded by one or more layers of flattened cells. The resemblance to ovarian primordial follicles was striking in-

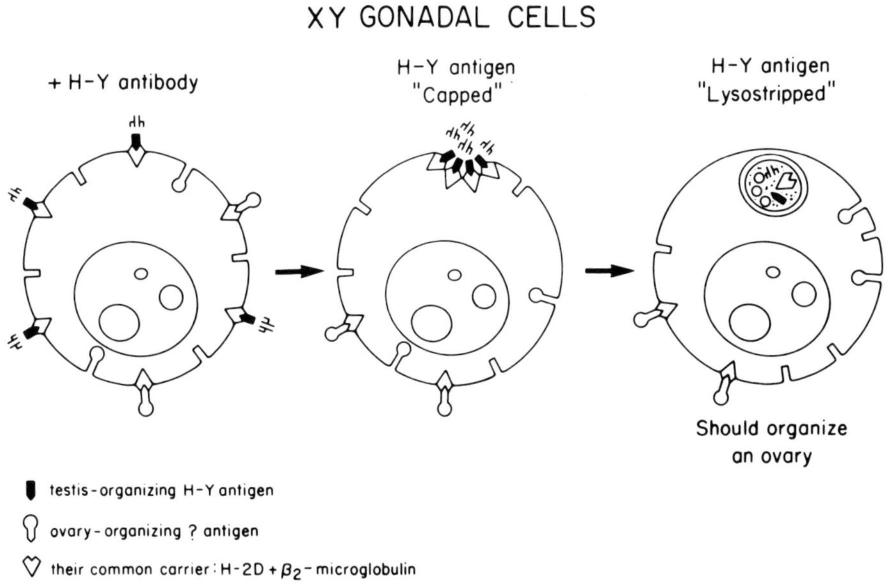

Fig. 11. Schematic illustration of the removal of H-Y antigen from the plasma membrane of newborn testicular cells by the use of excess H-Y antibody: H-Y antigen sites are first capped and then lysostripped. Although H-Y antibody is primarily IgM, in this scheme, each molecule is shown as an LH tetramer (IgG characteristic). This is merely for the sake of simplicity. It is assumed that the presumptive ovary-organizing antigen is constitutively expressed in male and female gonadal cells alike. Such constitutive production is implicit in the statement that the basic embryonic plan of mammalian gonads is inherently feminine

deed. While the presence of H-Y antigen in male gonadal cells is essential for their testicular organogenesis, its presence in male epidermal cells is obviously trivial. Indeed, male epidermal cells lysostripped of H-Y antigen, after the rotation culture, readily formed typical epidermis-like aggregates complete with what appear to be hair follicle-like structures. No hindrance was noted, thus confirming the specific testis-organizing role of the H-Y antigen (OHNO et al., 1978b).

If an inbred strain of rats, instead of mice, is used as a source of H-Y antibody as well as of newborn gonadal cells, the availability of a larger amount of H-Y antibody and of a greater number of gonadal cells permits the performance of Moscona-type reaggregation experiments on a considerably grander scale. The only drawback here is that no reliable cytotoxic assay method for H-Y antibody yet exists in the rat, so that the purity and specificity of H-Y antibody has to be assessed by one or the other histochemical method. Such experiments done by ZENZES et al., (1978) produced essentially the same result as described for the mouse. However, because of a longer period of rotation culture using a larger number of cells, the control culture yielded a testicular organ-like aggregate instead of short independent seminiferous tubule-like structures, while the H-Y antibody-treated culture produced an ovarian organ-like aggregate full of primordial follicle-like structures.

These two sets of reaggregation experiments have furnished the needed direct evidence in support of the proposed testis-organizing function of the H-Y antigen. It would appear then, that the hypothesis has been verified.

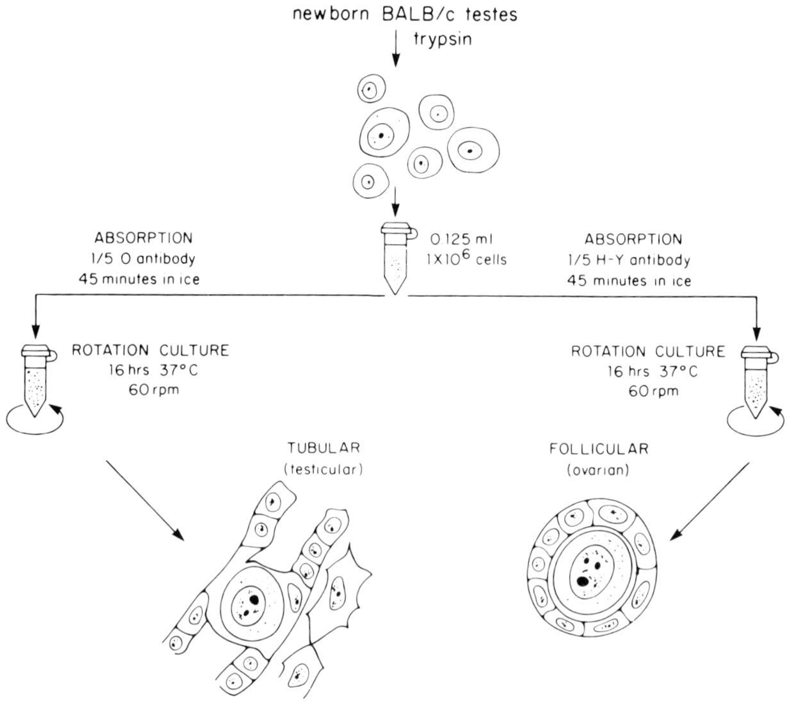

Fig. 12. Moscona-type reaggregation experiments starting from a suspension of free newborn testicular cells schematically explained

d) Polarized Distribution of the H-Y Antigen on the Plasma Membrane of Testicular Sertoli Cells and Underlying Mesenchymal (Basement Membrane) Cells

As far as I know, an attempt to map the distribution of various antigens on the plasma membrane was first made by BOYSE et al., (1968) on mouse thymocytes with regard to H-2D, H-2K, T1, Ly, and other antigens. They found that these antigens are not distributed at random but, rather, form distinct patches to produce a mosaic pattern. While the topographic distribution of H-Y antigen on the plasma membrane of male extragonadal somatic cells is of trival functional significance, that of male gonadal cells is an entirely different matter. Because H-Y antigen is apparently responsible for testicular organization, one hardly expects the homogeneous distribution of H-Y antigen on the plasma membrane of Sertoli cells or on their precursors, which are together with underlying cells engaged in seminiferous tubule formation. Some sort of polarized distrubution of the H-Y antigen is expected.

The first workable method for the histochemical visualization of H-Y antigen was developed by KOO et al. (1973). This technique utilized a rabbit hybrid antibody; one LH (light-heavy chain) dimer directed against mouse Ig such as H-Y antibody is polymerized with another LH dimer directed against either sheep red

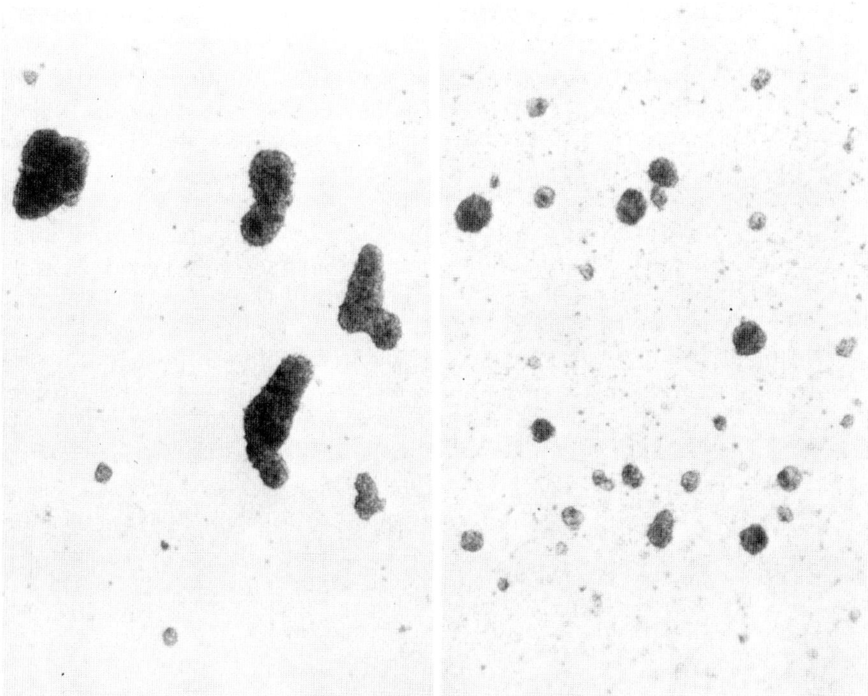

Fig. 13. Striking results of Moscona-type reaggregation experiments. Weakly magnified view of primarily tubular aggregates of a control rotation culture (*left*) is contrasted with that of numerous spherical aggregates that characterized the H-Y antibody-treated rotation culture (*right*). Tubular structures at *left*, although still short, already reveal the characteristic tendency of seminiferous tubules to twist and turn. lenses used: 2.5 x 10

blood cells for light microscop or tobacco mosaic viral particles for electron microscop. By this technique, they were able to show that the H-Y antigen of mouse spermatozoa is concentrated in the acrosomal region in which H-2 antigens have previously been localized. The known binding affinity of staphylococcal protein A to Fc regions of the IgG molecules (GHETIE et al., 1974) has also been utilized for the histochemical visualization of the H-Y antigen on male mouse lymph node cells (TOKUDA et al., 1977).

In our laboratory, we utilized a technique of Byzantine complexity developed by Dr. Klaus Bross of this Institute and slightly modified by Bruce Beutler, for our attempts to visualize H-Y antigen distributions on various component cell types of the newborn mouse testis. Various reagents with which free testicular cells, anchored to a siliconized glass slide via poly-*l*-lysine, were treated in succession, included: (1) mouse H-Y antibody, (2) rabbit antimouse Ig (G + M) antibody, (3) goat antirabbit IgG antibody, (4) rabbit antihorseradish peroxidase antibody, (5) horseradish peroxidase, and (6) diaminobenzidine, H_2O_2, and OsO_4. The most appropriate control was the substitution of mouse H-Y antibody with mouse anti-H-2 antibody directed against a wrong H-2 haplotype, i.e., anti-H-2^k antibody used against BALB H-2^d testicular cells. Most of the time, the experiment was a failure, because the control we used gave us some plasma membrane staining. However, on several occasions, the staining occurred only in the experimental group. On such rare occasions, we noted the uniform stain of the plasma membrane of primordial germ cells (Fig. 14, top). In sharp contrast, H-Y antigen stain on the plasma membrane of Sertoli cells showed a peculiar bipolar distribution; one stained area covered one-third to one-half of the circumference, whereas another small heavily stained knob was seen diametrically opposite from the center of a widely stained area (Fig. 14, bottom). The purification procedure for Sertoli and Leydig cells is discussed in Chap. 9. While similar bipolar distributions of H-Y antigen were seldom seen on the plasma membrane of Leydig cells, a small number of fibroblast-like elongated cells, presumably derived from the seminiferous tubule basement membrane, showed the extensive positive stain along only one of the two longitudinal cell surfaces. On the basis of the histochemical observations made on the plasma membrane of Sertoli and presumptive basement membrane cells, I have constructed a schematic drawing depicting the true organogenetic role of the H-Y antigen in seminiferous tubule formation (Fig. 15).

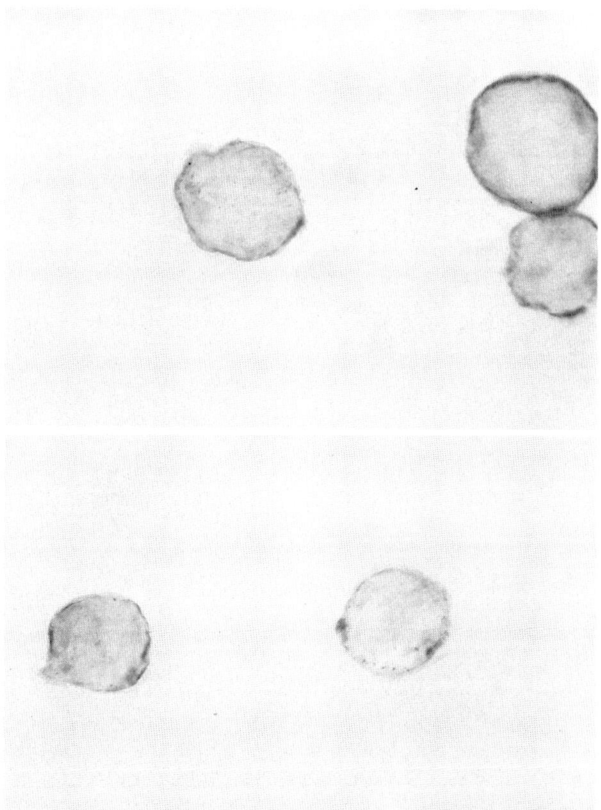

Fig. 14. Histochemical stain of H-Y antigen that ultimately utilized horseradish peroxidase. When the staining was specific, homogeneous distribution of the H-Y antigen sites on the plasma membrane of primordial germ cells is revealed (*top*). This is consistent with the notion that germ cells play a passive role in determining the fate of emerging embryonic gonads. H-Y antigen sites on the plasma membrane of Sertoli cells (*bottom*), in sharp contrast, reveal a unique bipolar distribution: H-Y antigen is concentrated along a wide area at the right of these two cells. However, a knob-like concentration of H-Y antigen is also seen at the left side of each cell

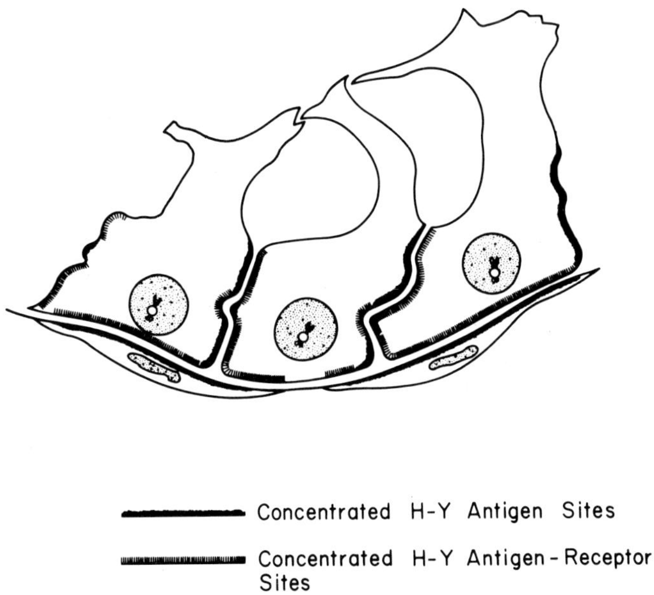

Fig. 15. Seminiferous tubule organization by mutually exclusive distributions of testis-organizing H-Y antigen sites and their specific receptor sites on the plasma membrane of Sertoli cells and their precursors. I believe that the mutual exclusiveness noted above is the reason for an apparently bipolar distribution of H-Y antigen sites. One-sided distribution of H-Y antigen sites on the plasma membrane of underlying mesenchymal cells is also essential for the formation of basement membrane. This scheme is based on my interpretation of histochemical observations described in the text and shown in Fig. 14

Chapter 8

The Developmental Strategy of Competitive Displacements and the Role of β_2-Microglobulin-H-2 or HLA Dimers in Organogenesis

The dominant role that plasma membrane components play in cell-cell interaction, and hence organogenesis, has long been suspected. Yet, at present, testis-organizing H-Y antigen constitutes the only example of a plasma membrane component to which a specific organogenesis function has been assigned. Accordingly, the significance of this antigen extends beyond its testis-organizing function, for it serves as a model for all other organogenesis-directing antigens that will be found in the future. No biological system can be error-free. Accordingly, accidental mishaps are bound to occur at various stages of development in embryos. Natural selection must have included various accommodations to either negate or minimize the effects of these mishaps as parts of the mammalian embryonic plan. It would be an ultimate folly, for example, to assign the task of being a primordium of one entire cell type to a single early embryonic cell, for the accidental death of that cell deprives an individual entirely of one particular cell type. Wisely, each developmental commitment in mammalian development is made by a group of cells and not by a single cell (McLaren, 1976). Similarly, accidental mix-ups between differently committed cells are bound to occur at territorial boundaries during the act of organogenesis. What if the diverticulum of a primitive gut, destined to be liver, accidentally incorporated a number of stray cells that had already made an initial commitment to be intestinal cells. Purely autonomous organogenesis by irreversibly committed individual cells would have produced an island of intestinal structure in the midst of liver. The very fact that such a mosaic organ is seldom, if ever, seen indicates the existence of a developmental strategy that avoids the formation of mosaic organs. A study on the fate of XX/XY mosaic or chimeric gonads reveals the nature of this developmental strategy, which is based on the principle of competitive displacements.

a) H-Y Antigen and the Fate of XX/XY Chimeric Gonads

The feat of producing one mouse out of two randomly fused blastocysts was originally accomplished by Tarkowski (1961). This technique has since been utilized extensively by B. Mintz, A. McLaren, R.L. Gardner, and W. K. Whitten, among others. Random fusions of two blastocysts should produce XX/XY sex chromosome chimeras 50 % of the time. Were XX and XY gonadal cells each to follow their respective inherent organogenetic dictates, the overall sex ratio of chimeric mice should be: one XX/XX female to one XY/XY male to two XX/XY true hermaphrodites. The fact is that true hermaphrodites seldom occur among chimeric mice. My literature survey revealed that of 550 described, only eight were true hermaphrodites: an incidence of 1.4%. A Curious dichotomy in reported sex ratios, however, cannot be ignored. When the data reported by TARKOWSKI and MCLAREN and their respective colleagues were combined, I found a sex ratio of 9 females (16.7%) to 41 males (75.9%) to 4 true hermaphrodites (7.4%). In sharp contrast, the combined data reported by MINTZ and GARDNER gave a nearly one-to-one sex ratio: 200 females to 192 males to 4 true hermaphrodites.

The above discrepancy is due mainly to a difference in strain combinations used. The first group used by TARKOWSKI and MCLAREN for blastocyst fusions consisted of two genetically very similar or compatible strains. For example, Tarkowski regularly used two congenic strains that differed from each other only with regard to T-6 marker chromosomes and a coat color gene. The second group of Mintz and Gardner, on the other hand, customarily used genetically distant strain combinations. WHITTEN (1975), among others, has pointed out that in strain combinations such as B10/BALB, one cell line is more vigorous and tends to outgrow the other, thus producing so-called unbalanced chimeras. Under the circumstances, it is no surprise if XX/XY chimeras always develop the sex of the dominant cell line. For example, if the cells of strain A tend to overgrow the cells of strain B, XX (A)/XY (B) chimeras will develop as females, whereas XX (B)/XY (A) chimeras will develop as males, thus yielding an overall sex ratio of one to one among chimeras of the A/B strain combination. Since naturally occurring XO/XY or XX/XY heterosexual mosaics usually develop from an XY zygote, the XO or XX cell line, being a derivative, is genetically identical to the ancestral XY line, except for the absence of the Y. It follows then that the finding of the first group (compatible) is far more relevant than that of the second group (dissimilar) to our understanding of the fate of naturally occurring heterosexually mosaic gonads. It would appear that heterosexual gonads consisting of a nearly one-to-one mixture of XX and XY cells most often organize testes, less often ovaries, and infrequently ovotestes. I should point out here that, as far as the laboratory mouse is concerned, a majority of the true hermaphrodites belong to the type that has a testis on one side and an ovary on the other (66.9%), whereas the type having a pair of ovotestes is the rarest (5.2%), as summarized by WHITTEN (1975). In man, however, the situation is somewhat different: The type having a testis or an ovary on one side and an ovotestis on the other appears to be most common (POLANI, 1970).

I have proposed the XY to XX transfer of H-Y antigen as the reason for testicular differentiation of XX/XY mosaic or chimeric gonads. By saturating the plasma membrane sites of neighboring XX cells with disseminated H-Y antigen, XY cells manage to entice XX cells in the same gonad to cooperate in the act of testicular organization (OHNO, 1976c). Although the ample amount of H-Y antigen found in exceptionally virilized testis-like fetal bovine freemartin gonads (that consisted essentially of XX cells), confirmed the postulated transfer of H-Y antigen to XX gonadal cells (OHNO et al., 1976), there is uncertainty about the source of gonadal H-Y antigen (see Chap. 10). Thus the study of chimeric mouse testes that consist roughly of a one-to-one mixture of XX and XY cells was deemed necessary. While the testes of the above composition are less likely to be found among XX/XY chimeric males of genetically distant strain combinations, such combinations enable us to exploit allelic differences at the H-2 and certain enzyme loci as tools to assess XX/XY ratios of various cell types.

Accordingly, we chose the BALB/C3H combination. All chimeric males produced by the laboratory of Dr. J. Melnyk of this institution were progeny tested by mating them to albino BALB females. As shall be discussed in the next chapter, XX primordial germ cells in the testicular environment are incapable of undergoing neonatal differentiation to become definitive spermatogonia. Accordingly, they become extinct at this stage. For this reason, XX/XY chimeric males of our strain combination, if they were fertile, sired either all agouti or all albino progeny out of albino BALB/c females. The agouti progeny were derived from C3H XY germ line, and the albino progeny from BALB XY germ line. Of several XX/XY chimeric males so identified by the progeny test, most revealed a great preponderance of XY cell line in all parts of their bodies, as expected. They were of little use.

Fortunately, one XX (BALB)/XY (C3H) male, while producing 39 agouti (18 males and 21 females) and no albino progeny, demonstrated more white than colored patches on his coat (Fig. 16). Subsequent analysis indeed revealed the presence of 50% or more of BALB XX cells in every somatic type examined. The XX/XY ratios of his spleen and tail epidermal cells were determined by cytotoxicity tests using anti-H-2^d antibody directed against BALB XX cells and anti-H-2^k antibody directed against C3H XY cells (Table 2). Testicular cells were first fractionated into germ cells and somatic elements by successive treatments with collagenase and then trypsin at two concentrations. While germ cells comprising 90% or more of the total were exclusively of the C3H XY line, as expected from the progeny test, the starch gel electrophoretic study of glucose phosphate isomerase revealed the XX:XY ratio among Sertoli and Leydig cells to be 1:1 (Table 2). H-Y absorption tests performed on these cell types revealed no evidence of the XY-to-XX transfer of H-Y antigen among spleen and epidermal cells (Table 1). This negative finding is relevant in interpreting the H-Y antigen expression reported on essentially XX cell populations of peripheral blood leukocytes and cultured fibroblasts of one human XX male who was actually an XX/XXY mosaic (WACHTEL et al., 1976 a), as discussed in Chap. 7. It may be that the XY-to-XX

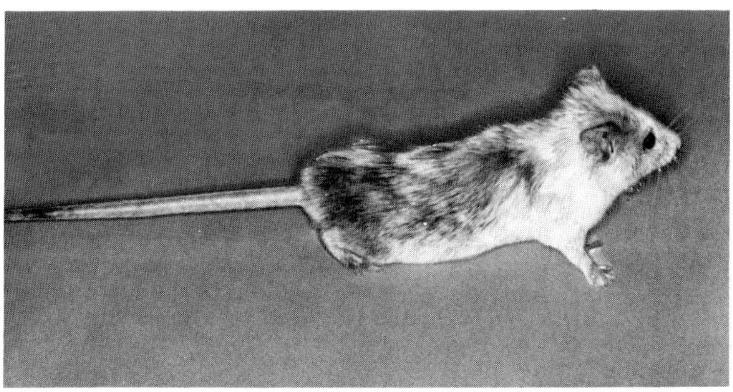

Fig. 16. Fertile XX (BALB)/XY (C3H) chimeric male mouse at 7 months of age. Coat color: albino [populated by XX (BALB) melanocytes] with scattered agouti [populated by XY (C3H) melanocytes] spots. See also Table 2

Table 2. The summary of our findings on an exceptional XX (BALB)/XY (C3H) male mouse. Two extragonadal cell types, spleen as well as epidermal cells, and testicular Sertoli and Leydig cells were used in nearly equal mixtures of XX and XY cells. The H-Y antibody absorption capacity of each cell type was expressed as a percentage of that shown by all male cells of the corresponding cell type of the parental strains (OHNO et al., 1978 a)

The XY→XX transfer of H-Y antigen among testicular Leydig and Sertoli cells but not among spleen and epidermal cells

	XX : XY	H-Y antigen (% of normal ♂)
Spleen cells	60 : 40 ($H\text{-}2^d$: $H\text{-}2^k$)	50% (absorption)
Epidermal cells	55 : 45 ($H\text{-}2^d$: $H\text{-}2^k$)	40% (cytotoxicity)
Testicular germ cells	0 : 100 (BALB GPI : C3H GPI)	100% (absorption)
Testicular Leydig + Sertoli cells	50 : 50 (BALB GPI : C3H GPI)	135% (absorption)

transfer of H-Y antigen among extragonadal somatic elements cannot occur because the disseminated H-Y antigen that they encounter is in association with β_2-microglobulin. Only free H-Y antigen is expected to demonstrate the binding affinity to the unoccupied β_2-microglobulin-MHC antigen dimer site on the plasma membrane. The situation found on testicular Sertoli and Leydig cells of this balanced XX (BALB)/XY (C3H) chimeric male mouse was very different from those found in his spleen and epidermal cells. Despite the fact that half of these testicular cells were BALB XX, their H-Y antibody absorption capacity actually surpassed that of normal males of either parental strain (Table 2). Thus, the reason that XX gonadal cells in a mosaic or chimeric gonad are often enticed to participate in testicular organogenesis can now be attributed to the XY-to-XX transfer of H-Y antigen. A more detailed description of this most informative XX/XY chimeric male mouse has been given elsewhere (OHNO et al. 1978a). While it presently appears that the H-Y antigen disseminated by neighboring XY cells is the sole source of this antigen found on the plasma membrane of XX cells that constituted the sexually mosaic or chimeric testis, an alternative possibility although unlikely, that XX gonadal cells inherently are capable of producing their own H-Y antigen, if properly stimulated, shall be discussed in Chap. 10. Because of the neonatal elimination of XX germ cells from the XX/XY testis, we were unable to witness the XY-to-XX transfer of H-Y on germ cells of this sexually mature XX (BALB)/XY (C3H) male. Were we to have studied him at the fe-stage, I am reasonably certain that the H-Y antigen would also have been found on the plasma membrane of XX primordial germ cells. It is worth noting that in the mouse differentiation from primordial germ cells to much smaller definitive spermatogonia invariably occurs neonatally (ROUSEN-RUNGE, 1964).

Although less frequent than XX/XY males, XX/XY chimeric female mice also have been identified. When fertile, they may ovulate XY oocytes (EVANS et al. 1977). It would appear that the reverse competitive displacement of testis-organizing H-Y antigen with a yet to be identified ovary-organizing antigen can occur on the plasma membrane of XY gonadal cells. The absence of H-Y antigen on the plasma membrane of XY ovarian cells, germ and soma alike, however, is technically hard if not impossible to prove by H-Y antibody absorption tests. Mouse ovaries are simply too small to supply the large number of cells ($40\text{-}80 \times 10^6$) required for the negative proof of their H-Y antibody absorption capacity. Nevertheless, it can be recalled from Chap. 7 that in the absence of H-Y antigen, XY gonadal cells of fertile XY wood lemming females readily organized the functional ovary (FREDGA et al. 1976: WACHTEL et al. 1976 b). Furthermore, in *in vitro* reaggregation experiments, testicular Sertoli cells lysostripped of their H-Y antigen behaved as though they were now ovarian follicular cells (OHNO et al., 1978b; Zenzes et al., 1978), as shown in Fig. 13.

The above-noted study on XX/XY chimeric mouse testes gave strong supportive evidence to the notion of competitive displacements of one organogenesis-directing antigen with another on the plasma membrane of engaged cells as the developmental strategy that mammals employ to avoid the formation of mosaic organs. The reason that XX/XY gonads show a far greater tendency to develop as a testis than as an ovary is self-evident. Both the experiments of nature that we witnessed in the wood lemming and *in vitro* reaggregation performed on newborn mouse and rat testicular cells have shown that XY gonadal cells too have the inherent inclination to organize an ovary, and it is the H-Y antigen that prevents this predisposition from manifesting itself. It is likely, then that the production of a yet to be identified ovary-organizing antigen is constitutive in both sexes. It follows that during the act of normal testicular organogenesis, XY gonadal cells have the need to displace their own ovary-organizing plasma membrane antigen with disseminated H-Y antigen. Obviously, this physiologic need to disseminate testis-organizing H-Y antigen during the normal course of testicular organogenesis gives XY gonadal cells a decisive advantage over XX gonadal cells when the two confront each other in the XX/XY mosaic or chimeric gonad.

b) H-Y Antigen and True Hermaphrodites

As far as etiology is concerned, the most readily understandable form of true hermaphrodites in the mouse are sex chromosome mosaics: X0/XY, XX/XY, XX/XXY etc. Very disparate XX/XY ratios between left and right gonads can easily explain the fact that, among mice, the most common form of true hermaphroditism is that of a testis on one side and an ovary on the other. One again sees the developmental strategy of competitive displacements at work. In addition, this form makes us realize the short-range effectiveness of disseminated H-Y antigen as a testis-organizing hormone (OHNO et al., 1976). H-Y antigen disseminated by one gonad is incapable of affecting the fate of another gonad on the other side *via* the blood stream. This short-range effectiveness of disseminated H-Y antigen also explains the formation of ovotestes.

Within an XX/XY gonad, an extreme local paucity of XY gonadal cells can result in the formation of ovarian tissue adjacent to the testicular one. The fact that sex chromosome mosaicism can even have a heritable basis has been shown by the study of the BALB/cWt strain by WHITTEN (1975). In this strain, a relatively high incidence of true hermaphrodites is associated with a markedly distorted sex ratio in favor of females: The incidence of females is 62%. It is the heritable mitotic instability of the Y chromosome during early cleavage divisions that causes a considerable proportion of the XY zygotes to become X0/XY mosaics. It would appear that many of them become normal females, thus contributing to an excess of females. Nevertheless, this is the cause of true hermaphroditism in the BALD/cWT strain.

Unfortunately, all forms of sex chromosome mosaicism can be held accountable as the cause for only a minority of the naturally occuring true hermaphrodites. For example, in Polani' s survey of human true hermaphrodites, sex chromosome mosaicisms were found in only 24.5% of the total, while 58.4% had the XX sex chromosome constitution, and the remainder, the XY (POLANI, 1970). I already noted in the previous chapter that every one of the small number of human XX true hermaphrodites subjected to the serologic study of the H-Y antigen typed as positive in the same manner as human XX males (WACHTEL et al., 1976 a).

It is probable that XX males an XX true hermaphrodites are two sides of the same coin. Indeed, an apparent autosomal dominant gene found in a family of cocker spaniel dogs produced both XX males and XX true hermaphrodites (SELDEN et al., 1978). In the goat, it is an autosomal recessive gene that produces XX males and XX true hermaphrodites (HAMERTON et al., 1969). A point of further interest concerning these cocker spaniels was that one H-Y antigen positive, true hermaphrodite with a pair of ovotestes functioned as a fertile bitch and produced a litter that included an XX male pup. It is of interest here to recall Whitten' s experience with his BALD/cWt strain. True hermaphrodites of this mouse strain, having a testis on one side and an ovary on the other, can function as fertile males upon removal of their ovary. By transplanting a removed ovary to a normal castrated female and then mating her to that unilaterally ovariectomized true hermaphrodite, he has, in fact, accomplished self-fertilization in the mouse (WHITTEN, 1975).

I shall end this section on true hermaphrodites by quoting the personal experience of S. S. Wachtel. He received a shipment of two separate botteles of cultured fibroblasts from a certain clinic with no pertinent information attached to them. The H-Y antibody absorption tests that he nevertheless performed revealed the first bottle to contain H-Y (+) fibroblasts and the second bottle, H-Y (-) ones. After a considerable time, he was informed that positive cells in the first bottle were derived from a testicular portion, and negative cells in the second bottle were from an ovatian portion of one human XX ovotestis.The strategy of competitive displacement is again in evidence. The reason that a gonad consisting entirely of H-Y antigen-positive XX cells develops as an ovotestis must lie either in the subnormal capacity of these cells to disseminate H-Y antigen or an abnormally prominent display of a yet to be defined ovary-organizing antigen on the plasma membrane. Either way, a pocket of H-Y antigen-negative gonadal cells may develop during testicular organization, which then organize ovarian tissue.

c) β_2-Microglobulin-MHC (H-2 of the Mouse and HLA of Man) Antigen Dimers as the Plasma Membrane Anchorage Site of Testis-Organizing H-Y Antigen

Discussions in the previous section made us realize that neither XY nor XX gonadal cells of mammals are irreversibly committed to their respective organogenetic destinies. When these two cell types are placed in proximity to each other, their

and SILMSER, 1955). While H-2 homozygous females consistently rejected isologous male grafts, H-2^k females did not. Yet, H-2^bH-2^k F1 females rejected H-2^k male grafts more vigorously than H-2b male grafts. The reason for the nonrejector status of C3H and other H-2^k strains became immediately obvious. Immune response (Ir) genes (Ia, Ib etc., of Fig. 17) residing within the H-2^k region of female responder T cells are not very competent in recognizing and responding to H-Y antigen when it is presented in conjunction with β_2m-H-$2D^k$ as well as β_2-m-H-$2K^k$ dimers by the plasma membrane of male target cells. Ir genes residing within the H-2^b region of female responder T cells, in sharp contrast, have no difficulty in recognizing the combination of H-Y and β_2-m-H2^k on the male target plasma membrane. More on the male target plasma membrane. More recent *in vitro* cell-mediated immune response studies on female T-cell killings of H-2 compatible male target cells revealed essentially the same thing in more sophisticated details (GORDON et al., 1975., GORDON et al., 1976., SIMPSON and GORDON, 1977).

The question then arose, Why does the female T-cell insist upon recognizing H-Y antigen only in conjuction with H-2 antigens? There were two obvious alternatives: (1) By physical association, H-Y and β_2-m-H-2D and/or β_2-m-H-2K dimers form hybrid antigens on the plasma membrane of male cells. (2) Each cytotoxic T cell is equipped with a set of two receptors: one for recognizing a specific antigen such as H-Y and the other for recognizing β_2-mH-2 antigen dimers. The second alternative postulates that in order to kill the target, both receptors of attacking T cells have to find properly matched antigens. The evidence that favors the first alternative over the second has already been presented in Fig. 9. It should be recalled that H-2 haplotypes determine the male target cell's cytotoxic sensitivity to H-Y antibody (SCHEID et al., 1972). Cytotoxicity tests for H-Y antibody do not include female T cells in the reaction mixture. In a very broad sense, H-Y antigen and β_2-m-H-2 antigen dimers can be considered as a hapten and its carrier. The H-Y antibody absorption test detects a hapten by itself, hence, the remarkable evolutionary conservation of H-Y antigen revealed by this test (WACHTEL et al., 1975a). To be cytotoxic, on the other hand, H-Y antibody has to find a hapten complexed with a carrier, hence, the observed influence of H-2 haplotypes on the cytotoxic sensitivity of male target cells to H-Y antibody (see Fig. 9). The notion of β_2-m-MHC antigen dimers serving as the plasma membrane anchorage site of H-Y antigen implies that H-Y antigen itself is not in direct contact with the plasma membrane of male target cells. Accordingly, H-Y antibody has to reach the target plasma membrane through a β_2-m-H-2 antigen dimer that lies under the H-Y antigen. One can easily imagine how conformational differences of underlying β_2-m-H-2 antigen dimers affect the cytotoxic effectiveness of H-Y antibody.

By the same token, one can imagine that the cytotoxic effectiveness of anti-H-2 antibodies would be hindered by H-Y antigen as it sits on the top of β_2-m-H-2 antigen dimers. H-Y antigen is but one of the presumably many (20 or so?) organogenesis-directing antigens. Nevertheless, the total number of organogenesis-directing antigen sites can never exceed the number of their anchorage sites. Furthermore, some organogenesis-directing antigens may show a preference toward β_2-m-H-2D antigen dimers, while others may prefer to associate with β_2-m-H-2K. All in all, there will always be empty plasma membrane anchorage sites, and the ratios between occupied and unoccupied anchorages sites may vary from one cell type to another. One expects the cell type with the largest proportion of unoccupied β_2-m-H-2 sites to be most sensitive to the cytotoxic effect of anti-H-2 antibody.

I believe the above to be the very reason for extraordinary sensitivities to the cytotoxic effect of anti-H-2 antibody displaed by circulating lymphocytes and other hematopoietic cells. Because these freely wandering cells do not engage in any sort of organogenesis *per se*, most of the β_2-m-H-2 antigen sites on their plasma membrane, being unoccupied, offer themselves as tempting cytotoxic targets to anti-H-2 antibody. In sharp contrast, any cell type that constitutes an integral part of the solid organ is expected to have a very small proportion of their β_2-mH-2 antigen dimers in the unoccupied state. Hence, the marked ineffectiveness of anti-H-2 antibody toward this type of target cells.

In Fig. 18, the cytotoxic sensitivity to anti-H-2^d antibody of BALB mouse spleen cells is contrasted with that of BALB epidermal cells. Spleen cells repre-

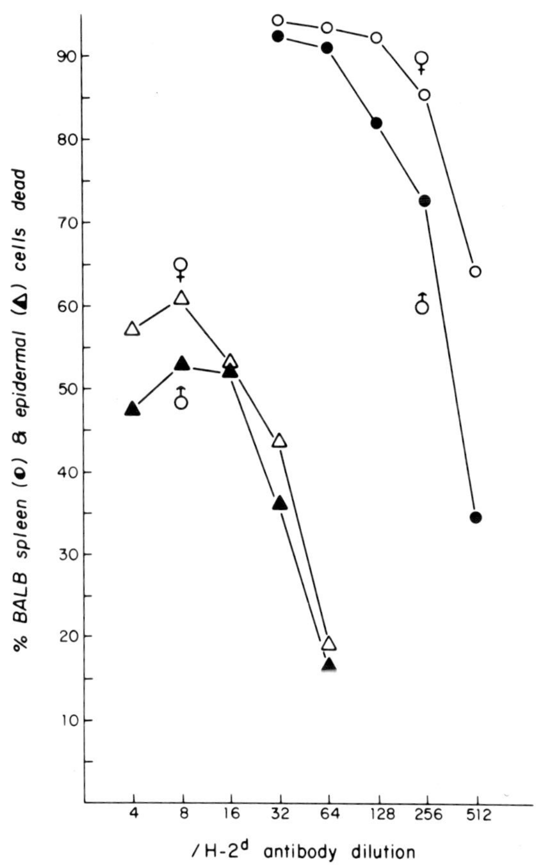

Fig. 18. Direct cytotoxicity tests using anti-H-2^d antibody in the presence of agarose-absorbed guinea pig complement. Extreme cytotoxic sensitivities of male (○) and female (●) spleen cells from adult BALB mice are contrasted with considerable insensitivities of male (△) and female (▲) epidermal cells of the same individuals

sent the hematopoietic cell types that are extremely sensitive, while epidermal cells represent the solid-organ-derived cell types that are relatively resistant. If the cytotoxicity of anti-H-2^d antibody on male BALB epidermal cells, shown in Fig. 18, is compared with that of H-Y antibody on the identical cell type shown in Fig. 8, it becomes clear that as far as this particular cell type is concerned, anti-H-2 antibody is no more cytotoxic than H-Y antibody. In this connection, a slight but remarkably consistent sexual difference in the cytotoxic sensitivity to anti-H-2 antibodies that we found on spleen as well as on epidermal cells should be noted (Fig. 18). An additional fraction of the β_2-m-H-2 antigen dimers on the male plasma membrane occupied by ubiquitously expressed but male-specific H-Y antigen, can readily explain slight, but consistently more resistance to the cytotoxic effect of anti-H-2 antibodies shown by male mouse cells.

Since the original demonstration by ZINKERNAGEL and DOHERTY (1974), it has been established that the T-cell killing of virally infected or transformed target cells is as H-2 restricted as the female T-cell killing of H-Y incompatible (male) target cells. Whether or not the observed H-2 restriction reflects the physical association between viral antigens and β_2-m-H-2 antigen dimers on the target cell plasma membrane has been tested by co-capping (SCHRADER et al., 1975) and co-lysostripping (HENNING et al., 1976) experiments. The rationale of these experiments is as follows.

If all the viral antigens, such as an envelope protein, gp70, of murine leukemia virus are in physical association with β_2-m-H-$2D^b$ antigen dimers on the plasma membrane of H-2^b tumor cells, the exposure to an excess amount of anti-H-$2D^b$ antibody, but not of anti-H-$2K^b$ antibody, followed by the exposure to xenogenic antimouse IG antibody should cause the simultaneous capping (see Fig. 11) of not only β_2-m-H-$2D^b$ antigen dimers but also gp70. Since capped antigens are subsequently consumed by the process of autophagocytosis, the above treatment should denude the tumor cell plasma membrane of not only β_2-m-H-$2D^b$ antigen dimers but also gp70. Consequently, for a period of several hours, treated tumor cells should remain insensitive, in the presence of complement, to the cytotoxic effect of anti-H-$2D^b$ as well as anti-gp70 antibody. While the results obtained by the above-noted authors were affirmative, the nature of the close physical association indicated by this type of experiment has remained unclear. β_2-m-H-2D antigen dimers and gp70 may, in fact, have remained as separate entities on the plasma membrane of virally transformed tumor cells, but the juxtaposed positions they occupy might have caused their co-capping and co-lysostripping.

It was felt that the proposed function of β_2-microglobulin-MHC antigen dimers as the plasma membrane anchorage site of testis-organizing H-Y antigen should be subjected to a more exacting test. As far as I am aware, somatic mutations that cause total deficiencies of either β_2-microglobulin or H-2 antigens are not known among mouse cell lines. In sharp contrast, mutational deficiencies of β_2-microglobulin have been identified in three or more human cell lines (NILSSON et al., 1974). The reason may lie in the fact that the human β_2-microglobulin gene is often involved in deletions due to its precarious position at the distal end of the long arm of chromosome 15 (ZEUTHEN et al., 1977). Furthermore, since the synthesis of HLA antigens by human cells is closely coupled with that of β_2-microglobulin, the total mutational deficiency of this microglobulin causes the complete disappearance of HLA antigens from the plasma membrane of mutant cells. However, when such a mutant cell is somatically hybridized to a β_2-m (+), HLA (+) partner, β_2-microglobulin, supplied by the latter, revives the expression of the hitherto silent HLA antigens by the former (KLEIN et al., 1977).

Thus, it was decided that the Daudi human male pseudodiploid Burkitt lymphoma lime, which is β_2-m (-), HLA (-), offered the best test of the proposal that human testis-organizing H-Y antigen utilizes β_2-m-HLA antigen dimers as its plasma membrane anchorage sites. In the total absence of its anchorage sites, the stable expression of H-Y antigen on the plasma membrane of Daudi should not occur. As controls of Daudi, we chose two other male pseudodiploid Burkitt Allymphoma lines both were β_2-m (+), HLA (+). Their respective numbers of H-Y antigen sites/cell were determined by an extensive series of H-Y antibody absorption tests using graduated numbers of test cells. Details of such H-Y antibody absorption tests were given in Chap. 6, Sect. b.

The number of test cells required for 50% absorption of male-specific cytotoxi city contained in 50 μl of standardized 1:4 diluted H-Y antibody was first determined on each cell line. The numbers, so determined, were inversely proportional to the numbers of H-Y antigen sites per cell. For β_2-m (+), HLA (+) Raji and Ramos, 4 x 10^6 cells sufficed for 50% absorption of the male-specific cytotoxicity of the standardized H-Y antibody (Fig. 10 and Table 3), whereas as many as 22 x 10^6 Daudi cells were required for the same task. Thus, it became evident that, in the total absence of its plasma membrane anchorage sites, the H-Y antigen level on the plasma membrane of Daudi cells had been reduced to a mere 20% of the β_2-m (+) male control level (Table 3). The same trend toward a markedly reduced H-Y antigen level was also observed on a male myeloma line, Simpsson 8226, which was partially deficient in β_2-m-HLA antigen dimers; 14 x 10^6 Simpsson cells were required for 50% absorption (Table 3).

Subsequently, somatic hybrids between β_2-m (-), HLA (-) Daudi, and a variety of β_2-m (+), HLA (+) cell lines were examined. As already noted, in these hybrids the expression of Daudi HLA plasma autigens, A 10 and BW 17, was revived. With restoration of its membrane anchorage sites, H-Y antigen levels of these somatic hybrids either returned to or actually exceeded the control H-Y antigen level. Thus, the H-Y antigen level of the Daudi x Raji 8A (o x o) hybrids became equal to that of Tetra Raji (a colcemide-induced tetraploid line of Raji), both requiring 4 x 10^6 cells for 50 % absorption (Table 3). The female x male somatic hybrids between Daudi and HeLa D98 were more informative. In these independently derived hybrids, H-Y antigen was supplied only by the Daudi nucleus. Yet DAD 1 and DAD 10 demonstrated remarkably elevated H-Y antigen levels; only 3 x 10^6 cells of the former and as little as 2 x 10^6 cells of the latter were required for 50 % absorption (Table 3). A somatic hybrid, HE HR-1/D98, between the β_2-m (+), HLA (+) male pseudodiploid Burkitt lymphoma P3HR-1 line and HeLa 98 served as an appropriate control of DAD 1 and DAD 10: 4 x 10^6 HE HR-1/D98 cells were required for 50 % absorption (Table 3). These observations left little doubt that the very low plasma membrane H-Y antigen level, demonstrated by Daudi cells, was due to the total lack of β_2-m-HLA antigen dimers as anchorage sites for H-Y antigen. Because H-Y antigen was not stably maintained on their plasma membrane, Daudi cells excreted an excessive amount of H-Y antigen into the culture medium. Details of these findings have been described elsewhere (BEUTLER et al., 1978).

Table 3. Summary of H-Y antibody absorption tests performed on Daudi β_2-m (−), HLA (−) human male pseudodiploid Burkitt lymphoma cells and their various β_2-m (+), HLA (+) controls. Female x male somatic hybrids between Daudi and β_2-m (+). HLA (+) HeLa D98 were particularly informative

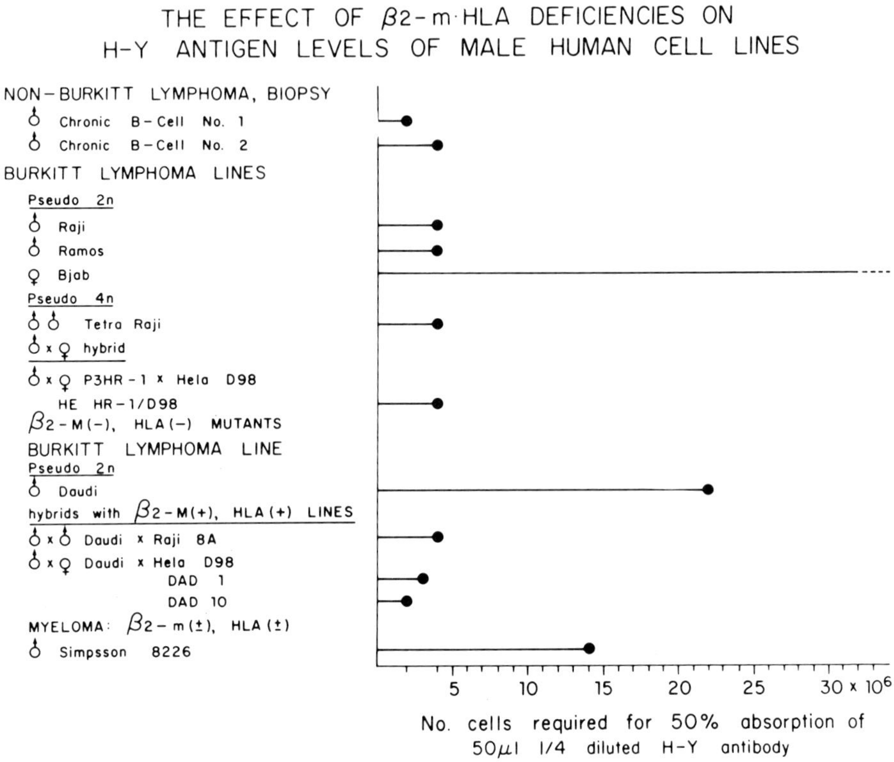

d) Why So Much Allelic Polymorphism at the Ubiquitously Expressed MHC Antigen Loci?

If the original function of β_2-m-MHC antigen dimers was to act as the general utility plasma membrane anchorage sites of all the organogenesis-directing antigens, one might think that mammals should have opted to maintain only one gene locus each for the β_2-microglobulin and the ubiquitously expressed MHC antigen. While there is apparently only one β_2-microglobulin locus, all the mammalian species that have been studied to date are endowed with two or more closely linked duplicated MHC gene loci: H-2D loci and H-2 K loci of the mouse, HLA-A and HLA-B loci of man. Having more than one MHC antigen loci creates a problem of specialization with regard to their plasma membrane anchorage function. In the mouse, for example, what if the testis-organizing H-Y antigen developed a preference for utilizing β_2-m-H-2D antigen dimers as its specialized anchorages sites, whereas the same sort of preference for β_2-m-H-2K antigen dimers was developed by an ovary-organizing antigen? Two opposing organogenesis-directing antigens can no longer compete against each other on the plasma membrane of gonadal cells. Accordingly, the organogenetic strategy of competitive displacements ceases to be operative. If there is to be a choice, a pair of competing organogenesis-directing antigens should always show the same preference, either for β_2-m-H-2D antigen dimers or for β_2-m-H-2K antigen dimers. On the other hand a liver-organizing antigen, for example, is not destined to contest its plasma membrane supremacy against a pair of gonad-organizing antigens, so that it is not obliged to utilize the same kind of anchorage sites used by the pair of gonad-organizing antigens. Thus, one sees the possibility of a division of labor among the anchorage sites. If the pair for gonadal organogenesis preferentially utilizes the type of dimer containing H-2D antigens for the plasma membrane anchorage sites, a liver-organizing antigen and its potential antagonist during the initial formation of liver primordium, an intestine-organizing antigen, can selectively make use of those containing H-2K antigens as their anchorage sites. In view of the ubiquitous expression of the H-Y antigen, which indicates a similar tendency on the part of other organogenesis-directing antigens, such a division of labor among their plasma membrane anchorage sites should serve to alleviate the hindrance of an organogenetic effort by the fortuitous presence of impertinent organogenesis-directing antigens. Indeed, we have seen that the presence of a rather large number of testis-organizing H-Y antigens on the plasma membrane of epidermal cells does not hinder the organization of epidermis by these cells (OHNO et al., 1978 b). I believe the above to be the evolutionary reason for having more that one MHC antigen locus in the mammalian genome.

Not only has the mammalian genome been endowed with two or more duplicated gene loci for ubiquitously expressed H-Y antigen, a very extensive allelic polymorphism characterizes each of these gene loci. Yet, amino acid sequence comparisons of the first 25 amino terminal residues of H-$2D^d$, H-$2D^b$, H-$2K^d$, and H-$2K^b$ polypeptide chains revealed not a single pair of locus-specific residues; the same can be said for HLA-A1, HLA-A2, HLA-B7, and HLA-B8 polypeptide chains (CUNNINGHAM, et al., 1977). If this trend continues for longer stretches of these polypeptide chains, H-2D and H-2K of the mouse, as well as HLA-A and HLA-B loci of man, can no longer be regarded as a pair of functionally differentiated loci. Instead, in the functional sense, a pair should be regarded as two extremely polymorphic copies of the same gene locus. In this event, a division of labor such as the plasma membrane anchorage sites of organogenesis-directing antigens just discussed, should be based on allelic instead of loci differences.

As discussed earlier in this chapter, on the plasma membrane of viral-infected or transformed cells, viral antigens also appear to utilize β_2-microglobulin-MHC antigen dimers as the plasma membrane anchorage sites. I observed previously that such competitive displacements of functionally important organogenesis-directing antigens, with their own antigens on the plasma membrane of host cells, constitute an integral part of the viral strategy; by so doing, parasitic viruses manage to sabotage the host cell's orderly function to gain an upper hand (OHNO, 1977b). Very extensive allelic polymorphism at H-2D and H-2K loci of the mouse as well as at HLA-A and HLA-B loci of man can be viewed as the host species' attempt to best cope with divergent pathogenic viruses. Indeed, when BALB/c x BALB/B (H-2^d/H-2^b) F1 mice were infected with Friend leukemia virus, infectious viral particles subsequently recovered preferentially contained H-$2D^b$ antigen exclusively (BUBBERS and LILLY, 1977). The subsequent study of

T-cell killings of Friend leukemia virus-infected H-2^d/H-2^b target cells indeed showed that in this attacker-target combination, H-2 restriction is caused exclusively by the preferential physical association between a viral antigen and β_2-m-H-$2D^b$ dimers on the plasma membrane of target cells (BLANK and LILLY, 1977). The binding affinity between a Friend leukemia viral (gp70?) antigen and β_2-m-H-$2D^b$ dimers must be one or two orders of magnitude higher than those involving three other types of dimers that are available: β_2-m-H-$2D^d$, β_2-m-H-$2K^d$, and β_2-m-H-$2K^b$. If a tighter binding between a viral antigen and β_2-m-MHC antigen dimers on the plasma membrane of infected or transformed target cells means more efficient handling of these targets by the host's cell mediated immune system, one can readily understand the persistence of H-2^b haplotype in a mouse population that is constantly exposed to Friend leukemia virus. I believe that herein lies a clue to our understanding of the emerging disease associations that involve an increasing number of HLA haplotypes of man.

As to the possible effect of allelic polymorphism of MHC loci on organogenesis, I have already noted that a majority of human true hermaphrodites are not sex chromosome mosaics (POLANI, 1970), let us imagine that a yet to be defined ovary-organizing antigen of man demonstrates an extraordinarily high binding affinity to β_2-m-HLA-B8 dimers. H-Y antigen-positive XX zygotes of all other HLA types would successfully organize testes, thereby becoming sterile XX males. However, in those that are either heterozygous or homozygous for HLA-B8 haplotype, disseminated H-Y antigen would encounter great difficulty in dislodging an ovary-organizing antigen from the plasma membrane of gonadal cells, thus developing as true hermaphrodites. I am confident that such an association between certain HLA haplotypes and true hermaphrodism of the nonmosaic types will be revealed in the future.

e) Identification of Disseminated Human H-Y Antigen in the Daudi Culture Medium

The fact that in the absence of the H-Y anchorage sites, β_2-m (-) HLA (-) Daudi human male Burkitt lymphoma cells maintain little or no H-Y antigen on their plasma membrane (BEUTLER et al., 1978) has recently been confirmed by others (FELLOUS et al., 1978). The latter authors also observed the co-capping of H-Y with β_2-microglobulin but not with H-2 antigens on male mouse cells. The observation that mouse H-Y does not co-cap with H-2 antigens was made previously (GEIBS et al., 1977). On the surface, it may appear that the H-Y antigen displaces H-2 antigens to form a dimer directly with β_2-microglobulin. In order to do so, however, the H-Y, by having a hydrophobic core must become an integral part of the plasma membrane, which would preclude its dissemination and therefore, its hormone-link role. The failure of H-Y to co-cap with H-2 antigens can easily be attributed to the difficulty that anti-H-2 antibodies have in coping with β_2-m-H-2 antigen dimers occupied by H-Y and other organogenesis-directing antigens (Fig. 18).

As reported at the 1978 Laurentian Hormone Conference, we have recently identified human H-Y antigen as the distinct molecular entity among Daudi excreted proteins. The molecular weight of its subunit is between 18,000 and

20,000. By the mean of interchain disulfide bridges, it appears to exist as an autotetramer, although the presence of autodimers and even autotrimers can not be excluded. As details shall be published in the next issue of Recent Progress in Hormone Research, I shall only describe the essence.

Exponentially growing Daudi human male Burkitt lymphoma cells were maintained in protein-free RPMI 1640 culture medium for the period of 16 h in the presence of tritiated lysine. During the above period, each one million Daudi cells excreted roughly 10 μg of proteins labeled at the ratio of 703 cpm/μg protein. For one series of experiment, labeled proteins excreted by the total of 150 million Daudi cells were pooled and concentrated. After removing free, unincorporated tritiated lysine by passing through Sephadex G-25 column. Sephadex G-200 eluates of these proteins were partitioned into four fractions according to their apparent molecular weights all the biological activities of H-Y antigen was recovered in Fraction I (void volume peak) representing only 14% of the Daudi proteins. For example, when 4 million bovine fetal ovarian cells were incubated with 2.2 ml of Fraction I solution containg 23.5μg of proteins, they absorbed 0.16μg of Daudi H-Y antigen on their gonad-specific H-Y antigen receptors and by so doing, these ovarian cells acquired the H-Y antibody absorption capacity nearly equal to that of bovine fetal testicular cells.

H-Y antigen subunit was identified by comparing the SDS gel electrophoresis profile of Fraction I with that from which H-Y antigen had selectively been removed by the exposure to a large excess of bovine fetal ovarian cells. If disulfide brigdes were broken by the mercaptoethanol pretreatment, the removal of H-Y antigen coincided with the disappearance of a molecular weight 18,000 to 20,000 peak. Without this pretreatment, a molucular weight 72,000 to 80,000 peak disappeared. The disappearance of the latter, however, was not as lear cut as that of the former. The fact that H-Y antigen eluted as the G-200 void volume peak reflects its tendency to form large aggregates in the concentrated state.

f) The Specific Receptor for H-Y Antigen Expressed by Gonadal Cells

The ubiquitous presence of H-Y antigen is the necessary but insufficient requirement for successful testicular organogenesis. In order to form the wall of seminiferous tubules, H-Y antigen sites on the plasma membrane of one Sertoli cell have to couple with their specific receptor sites on the plasma membrane of its immediate neighbors (Fig. 15). While the expression of H-Y antigen is ubiquitous in the male, that of the specific H-Y antigen receptor should be confined to gonadal cells. Nevertheless, the very fact that female XX gonadal cells by receiving H-Y antigen can be enticed to participate in testicular organogenesis in XX/XY mosaic gonads (Table 2) reveals that the expression of the gonadal H-Y antigen receptor is not male specific, female gonadal cells being endowed with this receptor (Ohno, 1976c). I have already noted that some of the XY women with pure gonadal dysgenesis express H-Y antigen although at somewhat subnormal levels. Their failure at testicular organogenesis might then be attributable to a mutational deficiency of the gonadal H-Y antigen receptor.

While H-Y antigen receptor sites on the testicular plasma membrane should naturally be in the fully occupied state by endogenous H-Y antigen, those sites on the ovarian plasma membrane are expected to be in the unoccupied state. The above was the very reason that enabled us to succesfully utilize bovine fetal ovarian cells for the identification of human H-Y antigen excreted by Daudi male Burkit lymphoma cells. Here, the gonad-specific H-Y antigen receptor should never be confused with the anchorage site of H-Y antigen provided by β_2-microglobulin-MHC antigen dimers. Because of a difference in their assigned functions, I expect the binding affinity toward H-Y antigen of the former to be several orders of magnitude higher than that of the latter.

After establishing the presence of free H-Y antigen in the epididymal fluid of adult male rats, MÜLLER et al., (1978) have indeed demonstrated the high affinity absorption of epididymal H-Y antigen by the ovarian, and to a lesser extent by testicular, membrane preparations. By contrast, those membrane preparations derived from extragonodal organs, such as liver, brain, spleen, and epidermis, demonstrated no appreciable affinity toward epididymal H-Y antigen.

The availability of tritium-labeled Fraction I Daudi proteins enabled us to obtain several pertinent information on the nature of the gonad-specific H-Y antigen receptor residing on the bovine ovarian plasma membrane. Knowing H-Y antigen to comprise 5% of Fraction I Daudi excreted proteins, and assuming the tetrameric form of the molecular weight 80,000 to be the natural state of H-Y antigen, it would be recalled that at the H-Y antigen concentration of 6.6×10^{-9}M, the saturation of all the available receptor sites still occured. The actual Kd of H-Y antigen toward its specific receptor is likely to be at least one order of magnitude less than the above. This indeed is a very respectable binding affinity. It would also be recalled that the saturation occured when 4 million bovine fetal ovarian cells absorbed 0.164 μg of Daudi human H-Y antigen. It would appear that each bovine ovarian cell is endowed with roughly 300,000 H-Y antigen receptor sites; again a very reasonable number.

Needless to say, only the induction of testicular organogenesis by H-Y antigen in solution constitutes the ultimate proof of this antigen's testis organizing function. When bovine XX indifferent gonads from embryos of 25 to 30 mm CR lenght were organ cultured for 5 days in the presence of 4.35×10^{-8}M Daudi H-Y antigen, the precocious formation of not only seminiferous and *rete* tubules but also of *tunica albuginea* indeed occured.

Chapter 9

Testis-Organizing H-Y Antigen and the Cell Lineage-Specific Antigen of Testicular Sertoli and Ovarian Follicular Cells: H-2 Restricted and Nonrestricted Killing by Female T-Cells of Testicular Sertoli Cells

Although male specific, H-Y antigen is, as far as we know, ubiquitously expressed in every somatic cell type of the mammalian male. At first glance, the assignment of a specific organogenesis-directing function to an antigen so ubiquitously expressed might seem rather absurd. A second thought, however, should make everyone realize that the omnipresent expression might actually be the hallmark of organogenesis-directing antigens. In order to direct organogenesis, an antigen responsible for it has to express itself before the scheduled commencement of that organogenesis. Indeed in the development of mouse embryos, gonadal differentiation does not begin until the 12th day (PETERS, 1970), yet H-Y antigen is first expressed ten days earlier in preimplantation male embryos of the eight-cell stage (KRCO and GOLDBERG 1976). Its ubiquitous expression may be viewed as a tolerable consequence of the need to express itself very early in embryonic development. The expression of H-Y antigen by male extragonadal somatic cell types is clearly as superfluous as the maintenance of the Y by the same cell types. Witness the fact that the male bandicoot, belonging to the two marsupial genera Isoodon and Perameles, eliminates the Y and acquires an X0 sex chromosome constitution for many of his extragonadal cell types (HAYMAN and MARTIN, 1965).

Yet one realizes that testicular organization involves not one but several different cell types. Accordingly the possession, by all, of the H-Y antigen, while an absolute prerequisite, is by itself insufficient for testicular organization. A set of additional plasma membrane antigens, each specific for a particular cell type, appears essential since somatic elements within the central gonadal blastema of an emerging male gonad must sort themselves out so that precursors of Sertoli cells can get together to form a wall of seminiferous tubules, while precursors of Leydig cells as groups stay outside the tubules. Such sorting out processes are likely to depend upon cell-cell recognition through the identical plasma membrane antigen. In the *in vitro* reaggregation experiments of gonadal cells noted earlier, testicular Sertoli cells, lysostripped of H-Y antigen, behaved as ovarian follicular cells (OHNO et al., 1978; ZENZES et al., 1978). Therefore, it occurred to us that testicular Sertoli cells and ovarian follicular (granulosa) cells might be endowed with the identical plasma membrane antigen, reflecting the fact that they belong to the same cell lineage.

We have seen that H-2 restricitions in T-cell killings of male target cells are a consequence of the physical association between H-Y antigen and β_2-microglobulin-MHC antigen dimers on the plasma membrane of male cells. The developmental strategy of competitive displacements, discussed previously in connection with the fate of XX/XY mosaic or chimeric gonads, obviously depends upon the functioning of β_2-microglobulin-MHC antigen dimers as the common plasma membrane anchorage sites of opposing organogenesis-directing antigens, e. g., testis-organizing H-Y antigen *versus* a yet-to-be-identified ovary-organizing antigen. The raison d'etre of cell lineage-specific antigens, on the other hand, is to function as the cell identity marker in cell-cell recognition. Thus, they should remain as permanent fixtures of individual cells instead of being disseminated and transferred to other cells. Accordingly, it is felt that, when the female T-cell killings of male target cells are based on a cell lineage-specific antigen, there should be no H-2 restrictions in their killings. With these considerations in mind, Ciccarese and I began a detailed immunologic study of testicular Sertoli cell plasma membrane (CICCARESE and OHNO, 1978).

a) Pure Sertoli Cells from XX, Sxr/-Male Mouse Testes

In the absence of the Y, an autosomal dominant Sxr gene of the mouse (CATTANACH et al., 1971) specifies H-Y antigen (BENNETT et al., 1977), thus producing sex-reversed XX, Sxr/-males. In their testes, XX primordial germ cells persist normally until birth. However, they are incapable of undergoing neonatal differentiation to become smaller definitive spermatogonia. Their total elimination occurs at this stage. LIFSCHITZ (1972) proposed that in normal XY spermatogonia, X inactivation occurs and that the mechanism is incapable of inactivating more than one X chromosome; hence no germ cells having more than one X chromosome can differentiate into definitive spermatogonia. A glance at Table 1 reveals that the mammalian X chromosome specifies a number of enzymes for cellular household chores. It is obvious that no cell can survive without the X. However, it has been known for a long time that definitive spermatogonia literally live sheltered by the large amount of cytoplasm of Sertoli cells. It may be that essential X-linked enzymes are supplied to spermatogonia by Sertoli cells. It is also of interest to note that while all other cell types of the mammalian body utilize the X-linked phosphoglycerate kinase (Table 1), male germ cells alone utilize an autosomally inherited isozyme (VANDEBERG et al., 1973); at least the X-linked PGK locus is indeed silenced in male germ cells. At any rate, the strongest support for Lifschitz' s proposal is found in the normally 0Y sex chromosome constitution of male germ cells found in the creeping vole, Microtus oregoni, as already noted (OHNO et al., 1963).

Whatever the reason, the absence of germ cells caused the seminiferous tubule to contain only Sertoli cells. Accordingly, prepubertal and early postpubertal testes of sterile XX, Sxr/-males (5-100 days of age) were an excellent source of pure Sertoli cells (Fig. 19, left). These testes enabled us to obtain 1.5-2.0 x 10^6 pure Sertoli cells per mouse by the following procedure. Bundles of seminiferous tubules gently teased out of each testis were first stripped of the attaching extratubular elements by a 0.5% collagenase treatment for 10 min at 37 °C. After washing a few times, denuded seminiferous tubules were subjected to a 0.5% trypsin treatment for another 10 min at 37° C. This yielded a suspension of free Sertoli cells (Fig. 20, left). As XX, Sxr/-males grew older, once prominent Sertoli-cell-only seminiferous tubules progressively collapsed, and the vacated spaces were filled in by masses of Leydig cells. Thus, these hypertrophied Leydig cells became the dominant testicular cell type (Fig. 19, right). A pure suspension of Leydig cells

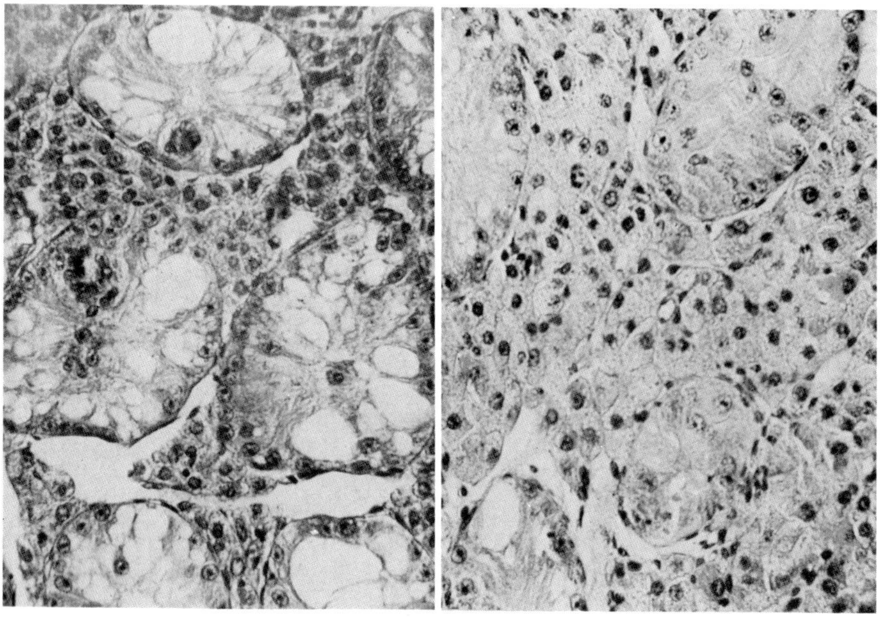

Fig. 19. Histologic sections of testes from XX, Sxr/- male mice. *Left*: From a 101-day-oldmouse. Sertoli cells – only seminiferous tubules are still prominent. A good source of Sertoli cells. *Right*: From a 182-day-oldmouse. Due to collapsing seminiferous tubules, hypertrophic Leydig cells dominate the field. A good source of Leydig cells. Lenses used: 45 x 10

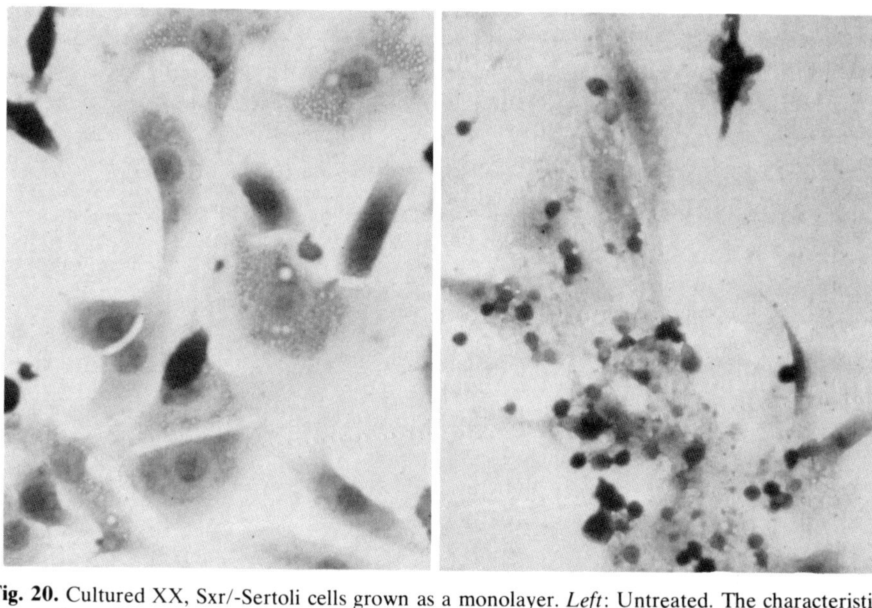

Fig. 20. Cultured XX, Sxr/-Sertoli cells grown as a monolayer. *Left*: Untreated. The characteristic morphology of a large round Sertoli cell nucleolus should be noted: one prominent nucleolus attached by one long, and one short heterochromatic body. *Right*: Under T-cell attack. Sertoli cells are being lysed by attached tiny T cells. Although there are crowds of T cells, actual killing is done by one or two attackers per target. Lenses used: 45 x 10

was readily obtainable from these older testes by the 0.5% collagenase treatment mentioned previously.

Our stock of mice, in which an autosomal dominant Sxr gene has been maintained together with two X-linked coat marker genes, Ta and Blo, initially went through six generations of brother x sister matings, and became homozygous for the H-2^k allele. Subsequently, two sublines, one homozygous for H-2^d and the other for H-2^b, were established by a once-only introduction to our stock of a BALB/c female for H-2^d, and of a C57B/6 female for H-2^b

b) Anti-Sertoli Antibodies Generated by H-2 Compatible Females Detect Two Plasma Membrane Antigens

H-2^d and H-2^k homozygous females of our mouse strains were immunized with three doses of 1.5-2.0 x 10^6 XX, Sxr/- Sertoli cells of the same H-2 type each, 8 to 9 days apart. A week after the last immunization, anti-Sertoli sera were collected from these females. These sera invariably were a mixture of two antibodies: H-Y antibody and the other antibody directed against the cell lineage-specific antigenic determinant shared by testicular Sertoli cells and ovarian follicular (granulosa) cells. How the above conclusion was deduced from the combinations of cytotoxicity and absorption tests can be seen in Table 4. In the presence of agarose-absorbed guinea pig complements raw anti-Sertoli sera were cytotoxic to male, but not to female adult epidermal cells, to testicular Sertoli cells of all ages, but only slightly so to adult Leydig cells, and not at all to newborn XY primordial germ cells. These sera were also cytotoxic to prepubertal ovarian follicular cells but not at all to adult luteal cells.

Although most cell types of the mammalian male readily absorb H-Y antibody raised in the mouse (WACHTEL et al., 1975a), this antibody is cytotoxic to only a very limited male cell type of the mouse, i. e., epidermal cells represent one of the

Table 4. Cytotoxic specificities of anti-Sertoli cell sera that contained H-Y antibody and antibody directed against a cell lineage-specific Sertoli-Follicular (S-F) antigen

	Testicular			Ovarian		Epidermal	
	primordial germ	Sertoli	Leydig	follicular	luteal	male	female
Unabsorbed	–	+++	+	++	–	+++	–
H-Y antibody removed by absorption with male BALB spleen or epidermal cells	–	+++	–	++	–	–	–
Further absorption ovarian follicular cells	–	–	–	–	–	–	–

+++: 21% – 27% corrected percent killings (see Fig. 21)
++: 15% – 20% corrected percent killings (see Fig. 21)
+: 1% – 5% corrected percent killings

few available cytotoxic targets of H-Y antibody (SCHEID et al., 1972). The male-specific cytotoxicity toward epidermal cells and a slight cytotoxicity toward testicular Leydig cells was indeed due to the presence of the H-Y antibody, for when raw anti-Sertoli sera were absorbed with an excess amount of either male epidermal cells (7 x 10^6 cells/50 μl of 1:4 diluted sera) or ample spleen cells (12 x 10^6 cells/the same amount), the preceding cytotoxicities were totally abolished (Table 4) while the absorption with female epidermal cells had no effect.

Once H-Y antibody was removed by the above procedure, what remained of the anti-Sertoli sera became highly specific. Among testicular elements, only Sertoli cells of all ages (5-100 days) were lysed by the antibody. The cytotxic sensitivity to this antibody was shown only by one other cell type: follicular (granulosa) cells obained from medium-sized follicles dissected out of prepubertal ovaries. Although the antibody was constistently more cytotoxic to testicular Sertoli cells than to ovarian follicular cells (Fig. 21), we believe that the difference was attributable to the relative impurity of the ovarian follicular cell fraction. Compared with the uniform appearance of Sertoli cell preparations under the microscope, our ovarian follicular cell fractions contained considerable proportions of spindle-

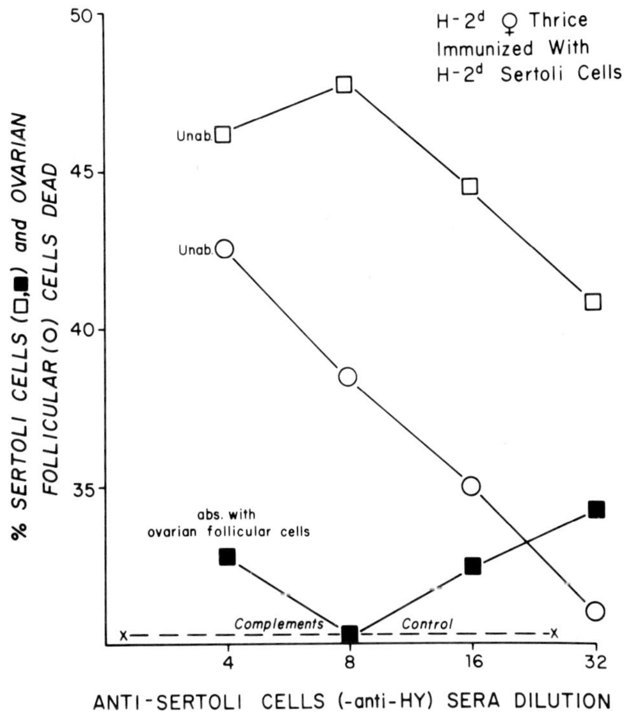

Fig. 21. Once H-Y antibody was removed by absorption using an excess number of either male epidermal cells or male spleen cells, the remaining anti-Sertoli antibody demonstrated cytotoxicity only to testicular Sertoli cells themselves and to prepubertal ovarian follicular cells. The absorption by ovarian follicular cells at the level of 12 x 10^6 cells/50 μl of 1:4 diluted antibody completely removed its cytotoxicity toward Sertoli cells. Thus, it was established that this antibody detects the identical or very similar antigenic determinant on the plasma membrane of testicular Sertoli cells and ovarian follicular cells

shaped fibroblast-like cells and rectangular (theca?) cells to which the antibody was not cytotoxic. The indication that the plasma membrane of testicular Sertoli cells and ovarian follicular cells possesses an identical or very similar antigenic determinant or determinants was further confirmed by the absorption test. When anti-Sertoli sera, from which H-Y antibody had been removed, were further absorbed with prepubertal ovarian follicular cells a t the level of 12 x 10^6 cells/50 μl of 1:4 diluted antibody, no residual cytotoxicity toward testicular Sertoli cells remained (Fig. 21 and Table 4).

In fact, doubly absorbed (first with male spleen or epidermal cells and then with ovarian follicular cells) anti-Sertoli sera demonstrated no cytotoxicity to any of the cell types listed in Table 4. Thus, the immunization of H-2 compatible female mice with XX, Sxr/- testicular Sertoli cells provoked the production of two antibodies from female responder B cells: One was directed against testis-organizing H-Y antigen, while the other recognized the cell lineage-specific antigen that marks testicular Sertoli cells and ovarian follicular cells as being derived from the same cell lineage.

Of course, this is not to suggest that these two are the only antigenic determinants on the plasma membrane of testicular Sertoli cells. Indeed, xenogenic antibodies such as rabbit and mouse Sertoli antibodies appear to recognize a great variety of antigens that are difficult to sort out. At any rate, within the confines of H-2 compatible systems the two presently identified appeared to be displayed most conspicuously on the plasma membrane of testicular Sertoli cells. It is fortunate that these two plasma membrane antigens appear most pertinent to testicular organogenesis.

Needless to say, the anti-Sertoli-follicular cell lineage-specific antibody was an autoantibody as far as immunized female mice were concerned. Obviously, histologic studies of immunized ovaries are necessary as well as breeding tests of immunized females. Our preliminary impression, however, is that this cell lineage-specific antigen on the plasma membrane of ovarian follicular cells rapidly disappears after puberty. It is for this reason that adult H-2 compatible females are able to generate an antibody directed against this self antigenic determinant. Whether the same antigenic determinant found on the plasma membrane of XX, Sxr/- testicular Sertoli cells can also be found on normal adult XY Sertoli cells has not yet been determined. In the normal adult testis, all the somatic elements together comprise little more than 5% of the total, and this makes it difficult to obtain a reasonably pure preparation of XY Sertoli cells. Anti-Sertoli antibody, however, was cytotoxic to a crude fraction of juvenile XY Sertoli cells. There remains little doubt that the presently identified Sertoli-follicular cell lineage-specific antigen is the normal plasma membrane component of testicular Sertoli cells, at least in the earlier stages of their development.

c) Two Plasma Membrane Antigens and H-2 Restricted Versus Unrestricted Lysis of Testicular Sertoli Cells by Doubly Primed Female T-Cells

Lymphocytes of all types are present in males and females alike. Accordingly, on the plasma membrane of syngeneic male spleen cells, female B and T cells recognize only one antigen as alien and that antigen has to be H-Y antigen. We have already noted that cytotoxic female T cells treat H-Y antigen in exactly the same manner as they treat viral antigens, so that lysis by primed T cells of H-Y incompatible target cells is H-2-restricted in the mouse as is lysis of virally infected or transformed target cells (GORDON et al., 1975; GORDON et al., 1976; SIMPSON and GORDON, 1977).

The developmental strategy of competitive displacements, already discussed, required testis-organizing H-Y antigen to function as a short-range organogenesis-directing hormone when the need did arise. For this reason, H-Y and possibly all other organogenesis-directing antigens utilize β_2-microglobulin-MHC antigen dimers as their plasma membrane anchorage sites. In the mouse, this physical association between H-Y and β_2-microglobulin-H-2 antigen dimers on the plasma membrane of male targets can be thought of as the cause of H-2 restrictions in lysis by cytotoxic female T cells.

We already noted that on the plasma membrane of testicular Sertoli cells, H-2 compatible female B cells recognized not only the H-Y antigen but also the Sertoli-follicular cell lineage-specific antigen. Thus, we can reasonably expect that H-2 compatible female T cells, if properly primed, would also recognize the same set of two antigens on the plasma membrane of target Sertoli cells. The latter antigen is likely to serve as the cell identification marker by which like cells can recognize each other. Thus, their role seems to dictate that such an antigen must exist as a nontransferable, integral component of the plasma membrane. No physical association with β_2-microglubulin-H-2 antigen dimers is expected on the plasma membrane of Sertoli cells. It follows then that lysis of target Sertoli cells by primed female T cells should show no H-2 restrictions if directed against the Sertoli-follicular cell lineage-specific antigen.

To study this problem, H-2 compatible female T cells were doubly primed in the following manner (CICCARESE and OHNO, 1978). From each of the H-2 compatible female mice that had been thrice immunized with XX, Sxr/- testicular Sertoli cells, the spleen was removed when the mouse was killed for the collection of anti-Sertoli antibodies, and a T-cell-enriched, was obtained by the nylon wool column filtration method (JULIUS et al., 1973). The 10-20 x 10^6 presensitized female T cells recovered from each spleen were then sensitized against the same target once again by culturing them together with 2 x 10^6 freshly prepared testicular Sertoli cells for 5 days. Doubly primed (thrice *in vivo* and once *in vitro*) female T cells were then used as attackers and mixed with freshly prepared Sertoli cells at the usual attackers-to-target ratio of 4 : 1, and the extent of lysis of target cells was monitored after allowing the attack to continue for 2.5 h; always two controls were used: (1) target Sertoli cells incubated alone; and (2) the 4 : 1 attacker-to-target mixture in which unprimed virgin female T cells of the same H-2 type were used as attackers. Of the two, the latter was a more appropriate control.

In the reaction mixture, the very large, rather flat Sertoli target cells were unmistakably distinct from the tiny attacking T lymphocytes. This enabled us to witness the actual killing by doubly primed T cells of target Sertoli cells under the microscope. Surprisingly, unprimed virgin female T cells of the control mixture readily attached themselves to the plasma membrane of Sertoli cells. However, such attachments caused no death of targets even when the large cell surface of a single Sertoli cell was literally saturated with 40 or more small lymphocytes attached to it. In sharp contrast, doubly primed female T cells were extremely efficient killers of Sertoli cells in the H-2 restricted as well as unrestricted situation. Lysis of a huge Sertoli cell was often caused by the attachment of only one or two tiny T cells. Under the attack, the large Sertoli cell cytoplasm literally boiled as it became progressively vacuolated. Then, the nucleus suddenly became pale and swollen. An individual killing took no more than one hour. Although 20 or more T cells were often found in the close vicinity of a target Sertoli cell, the actual killing always appeared to have been done by only one or two of them (Fig. 20, right). No doubt, the observed efficacy of individual cytotoxic T cells was the very reason that, despite a great difference in their sizes, the near maximal killing was already attained at an attacker-to-target ratio of 3:1 (Fig. 22).

Since Sertoli cells as targets were so distinct from attacking female T cells, the extent of lysis of attacked Sertoli cells was easily determined by the conventional trypan blue dye exclusion test routinely used for the cytotoxicity test of humoral antibodies (Fig. 22). In this type of *in vitro* T cell killing test, the corrected percent lysis value was determined by the following formula:

$$\text{Corrected percent lysis} = 100 \cdot \frac{\text{experimental dead cell \%} - \text{control dead cell \%}}{100 - \text{control dead cell \%}}$$

The same formula was also applied in compiling the results of cytotoxicity and absorption tests performed on anti-Sertoli antibodies (Table 4). In the case of humoral antibody cytotoxicity tests, control dead cell % meant complement control dead cell %.

We expected that if the double priming (thrice *in vivo* and once *in vitro*) by XX, Sxr/- testicular Sertoli cells generated cytotoxic female T cells directed exclusively against H-Y antigen, such T cells should lyse Sertoli cells as well as male spleen cells in the equally H-2 restricted manner. Conversely, if the doubly primed female T cell's wrath was directed solely against the Sertoli-follicular cell lineage-specific antigen, such T cells should show no cytotoxicity toward male spleen cells of any H-2 type, whereas they should readily lyse testicular Sertoli cells and ovarian follicular cells with equal ease, most likely in H-2 unrestricted manners. To test the preceding expectation, it was necessary to offer non-Sertoli cells of the above types to doubly primed female T cells as targets. Since these other target cells were not readily distinguishable from attacking T cells by their appearance, the extent of their lysis had to be measured by the ^{51}Cr (radioactive chromium) release test (GORDON et al., 1975). Unfortunately, most of our Sxr stock of mice, being either H-2^k or H-2^d homozygous, proved to be the least desirable strains in which to generate female cytotoxic T cells directed against H-Y antigen on the plasma membrane of male spleen cells (GORDON et al., 1975; GORDON et al., 1976; SIMPSON and GORDON, 1977). Indeed, H-2^d and H-2^k homozygous female T cells of our Sxr stock, when doubly primed with male

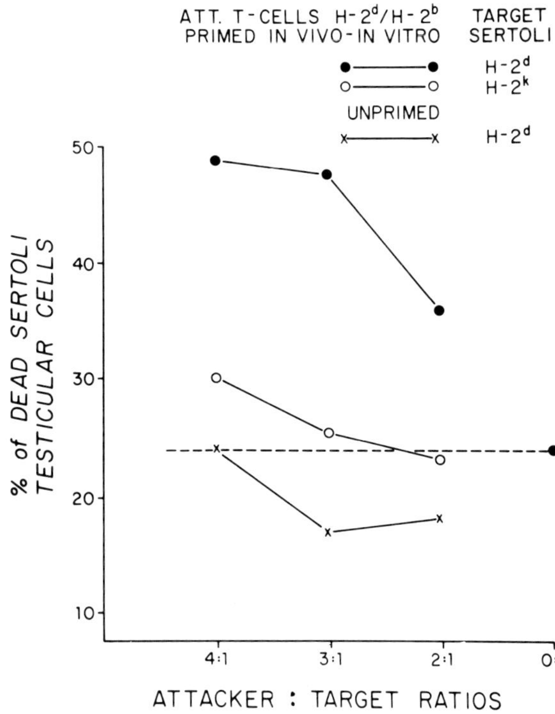

Fig. 22. H-2 restricted lysis of XX, *Sxr*/- testicular Sertoli cells by H-2^d/H-2^b (BALB/B6) F_1 female T cells doubly primed with male F_1 H-2^d/H-2^b spleen cells. Compatible H-2^d but not incompatible H-2^k Sertoli cells were lysed. Target nuclei stained with trypan blue were scored as lysed cells. An attacker-to-target ratio of 3:1 already resulted in the near maximal killing of H-2 compatible Sertoli cells. At the 4:1 ratio, the experimental killing of H-2^d targets was 47.5%, whereas the corresponding control value by unprimed virgin female T cells was 23.8%. Thus, using the formula shown in the text, the corrected percent lysis of H-2^d Sertoli cells was determined as 31.1%, whereas the corrected percent lysis of H-2^k Sertoli cells at the 4:1 ratio was 0.8%. Thus, in the first line of Table 5, the first value was scored as +++, and the second value as -

spleen cells of the same H-2 type, seldom caused significant lysis of H-2 compatible male spleen cells offered as targets. When the same priming was done by testicular Sertoli cells, however, these H-2^d as well as H-2^k female T cells readily lysed testicular Sertoli cells. Furthermore, when the Sertoli cell-killing was H-2 restricted, these T cells also lysed male spleen cells offered as targets, also in the H-2 restricted manner (Table 5).

There is little doubt that H-Y antigen sites are far more prominently displayed on the plasma membrane of testicular Sertoli cells than on those of male spleen cells. For example, we routinely attempt to produce H-Y antibody by five weekly injections of 5-20 x 10^6 syngeneic male spleen cells each. Yet by this procedure, only 25% of the immunized females yield H-Y antibody of a workable strength. In sharp contrast, a mere three consecutive injections of 1.5-2.0 x 10^6 testicular Sertoli cells unfailingly provoked each immunized female to produce potent H-Y antibody (Table 4).

We wanted to see if female T cells, directed exclusively against H-Y antigen, could lyse testicular Sertoli cells, and if they did, whether or not such lysis is H-2

Table 5. Two antigens on the plasma membrane of Sertoli cells and H-2 restricted and unrestricted lysis by H-2 compatibly primed female T cells

Premid with	Responder ♀ T cells	Target cells		
		H-2 type	Lysis	H-2 restriction
♂ spleen cells			Sertoli cells	
H-2^{d}/H-2^{b}	H-2^{d}/H-2^{b}	H-2^{d}	+++	yes
		H-2^{k}	–	
♂ spleen cells			Sertoli cells	
H-2^{d}/H-2^{b}	H-2^{d}/H-2^{b}	H-2^{d}	++	yes
		H-2^{k}	–	
Sertoli cells			Sertoli cells	
H-2^{d}	H-2^{d}	H-2^{d}	++++	
		H-2^{k}	±	
			♂ spleen cells	yes
		H-2^{d}	+	
		H-2^{k}	–	
			♀ spleen cells	
		H-2^{d}	–	
Sertoli cells			Sertoli cells	
H-2^{k}	H-2^{k}	H-2^{k}	+++	
		H-2^{d}	+++	
		H-2^{b}	+	no
			♂ spleen cells	
		H-2^{k}	–	
		H-2^{d}	–	
			♀ follicular cells	
		H-2^{d}	+	
Sertoli cells			Sertoli cells	
H-2^{d}	H-2^{d}	H-2^{d}	++	
		H-2^{k}	++	yes
			♂ spleen cells	&
		H-2^{d}	+	no
		H-2^{k}	–	
		H-2^{d}/H-2^{k}	+	
			♀ spleen cells	
		H-2^{d}	–	

Attacker-to-target ratio = 4 : 1

++++: 41%–46% corrected percent lysis
+++: 31%–40% corrected percent lysis
++: 21%–30% corrected percent lysis
+: 11%–20% corrected percent lysis
±: 5%–10% corrected percent lysis

restricted. This kind of female T cell can be generated by priming it with syngeneic male spleen cells. In view of the inadequacy of $H\text{-}2^d$ and $H\text{-}2^k$ homozygous strains for this purpose, we opted to sensitize BALB/B10 ($H\text{-}2^d/H\text{-}2^b$) F1 females with syngeneic F1 male spleen cells. Although GORDON et al., (1977) showed that BALB/B10 ($H\text{-}2^d/H\text{-}2^b$) F1 female T cells sensitized with syngeneic F1 male spleen cells while cytotoxic to F1 as well as to $H\text{-}2^b$ male spleen cells offered as targets, did not lyse $H\text{-}2^d$ male spleen cells, our doubly primed $H\text{-}2^d/H\text{-}2^b$ female T cells readily lysed compatibile $H2^d$ testicular Sertoli cells, but not incompatible $H\text{-}2^k$ Sertoli cells (Fig. 22 and the top two lines of Table 5). These findings thus established that H-Y antigen is the cause of H-2 restricted killing of testicular Sertoli cells by female T cells.

Three kinds of responses were noted when using $H\text{-}2^d$and $H\text{-}2^k$ female T cells of our Sxr stock were doubly primed with H-2 compatible testicular Sertoli cells. The third line from the top of Table 5 exemplifies the situation in which the cytotoxicity of doubly primed female T cells was directed exclusively toward H-Y antigen. As already noted, these T cells lysed both XX, Sxr/- Sertoli cells and XY male spleen cells in the H-2 restricted manner. The fourth line of Table 5, on the other hand, illustrates the alternate situation in which female T cells elected to ignore H-Y antigen all together and directed their entire attention to the Sertoli-follicular cell lineage-specific antigen. This type of female T cell was not at all cytotoxic to male spleen cells, even if H-2 compatible. Instead, they indiscriminately lysed Sertoli cells unrestricted by their H-2 types. They also lysed ovarian follicular cells. The third response exemplified in the bottom line of Table 5 was an obvious combination of these two. Accordingly, their killing of male spleen cells was H-2 restricted, whereas they indiscriminately lysed Sertoli cells unrestricted by H-2.

It appears that within the confines of H-2 compatibility, both B and T lymphocytes of the female immune system recognized the identical set of two antigens on the plasma membrane of testicular Sertoli cells: (1) ubiquitously expressed H-Y antigen and (2) the cell lineage-specific antigen which testicular Sertoli cells share with ovarian follicular cells of the female. While H-Y and possibly other organogenesis-directing antigens have the developmentally compelling reason to utilize β_2 -microglobulin-MHC antigen dimers as their plasma membrane anchorage sites, cell lineage-specific antigens, such as the presently found Sertoli-follicular antigen, have no need to do so, for their function apparently is to serve as the plasma membrane identification markers in cell-cell recognition. It stands to reason then that H-2 restriction in killing of testicular Sertoli cells by female T cells occured only when the attackers' wrath was directed exclusively toward H-Y antigen.

d) Relevance of These Two Antigens to Testicular Organogenesis

Inasmuch as H-Y antigen is possessed by all the cell types of developing male gonads, testicular organogenesis under the direction of H-Y antigen has to depend upon a set of cell type-specific antigens that enable individual cells of the same lineage to identify each other. One such antigen presently identified on the plasma membrane of Sertoli cells was also identified on ovarian follicular cells.

Such a sex-independent expression of the cell lineage-specific antigen by gonadal cells appears to form a foundation that enables ubiquitously expressed H-Y antigen to play such a pivotal role in the primary (gonadal) sex determination of mammals. Indeed, *in vitro* reaggregation experiments mentioned in Chap. 7 have shown that when lysostripped of their H-Y antigen, testicular Sertoli cells behave as though they are ovarian follicular cells (OHNO et al., 1978b; ZENZES et al., 1978).

The above experiment as well as the natural occurence of fertile XY females that are H-Y antigen negative in the wood lemming (FREDGA et al., 1976; WACHTEL et al., 1976b) also indicates the sex independent or bisexual expression of H-Y antigen's principal rivals; an ovary-organizing plasma membrane antigen and its membrane-bound receptor. Yet, if the expression of the H-Y antigen receptor were as male-specific as H-Y antigen itself, H-Y antigen would have to share the master regulatory role with its receptor. As we now know, the H-Y antigen receptor is expressed only by gonadal cells, but of both sexes.

From the above, we come to realize that there has been no *a priori* evolutinary reason for H-Y antigen being made of no more than 200 amino acid residues to play the pivotal role in the primary sex determining mechanism of mammals. It is the sex independent or bisexual expression of all other plasma membrane components involved in gonadal organogenesis that elevated the male-specifically expressed H-Y antigen to the top of the vast regulatory hierarchy.

Chapter 10

Why Are a Number of Unlinked Genes Involved in H-Y Antigen Expression ?

The master regulatory gene that occupies the very top of a regulatory hierarchy, by its very definition should not be under the regulatory influence of any other gene. It is true that by forming a feedback loop, any gene can assume the dual role of being at once the regulator and the regulated. This form of genetic regulatory system, however, is likely to operate at the periphery of a given regulatory hierarchy. Organogenesis being one of the earlier events of ontogeny, the role of organogenesis-directing antigen is to trigger the sequential activation of subsidiary regulatory systems, some of which may form feedback loops.

Since the egg cytoplasm of mammals is not particularly large, maternally stored proteins and *messenger* RNAs are quickly exhausted soon after fertilization. Accordingly, those genes in the zygotic nucleus required for various cellular household chores are mobilized for active duties within a few days after fertilization. The fact that H-Y antigen also becomes detectable for the first time in male preimplantation embryos of the 8-cell stage (2-2.5 postcoital days), along with a host of household enzymes, suggests that the activation of H-Y structural gene in zygotic development does not depend upon a special triggering mechanism. Furthermore, the subsequent expression of H-Y is ubiquitous. Indeed, befitting its primary regulatory role, the H-Y structural gene appears to be under the control of neither temporal nor cell type-specific regulatory systems. In addition, testicular organogenesis, as well as H-Y antigen expression, is not influenced by sex steroids. Female rabbits with extremely high titers of anti-testosterone antibodies can be made pregnant. Although remarkably high circulating testosterone levels are maintained by the mother aswell as by the fetuses, this antibody-bound testosterone is not at all accessible to fetal androgen-target organs. As a result, XY male embryos fail to develop most of the extragonadal masculine characteristics. Yet even such extreme testosterone deprivation does not affect testicular organogenesis in the slightest (BIDLINGMAIER et al., 1977). Similarly, the mutationally caused total insensitivity to testosterone does not affect the H-Y antigen level of testicular feminized XY (*Tfm*/Y) mice (BENNETT et al., 1975).

Inasmuch as the expression of testis organizing H-Y antigen by mammalian males is constitutive as well as ubiquitous, one would have thought that the simple evolutionary decision of endowing the male-specific Y chromosome with the H-Y structural gene should have sufficed for establishment of the mammalian primary sex-determining mechanism. Yet fertile XY wood lemming females have shown us that in the presence of an X-linked mutation, the normal Y chromosome became powerless with regard to its testic-organizing capacity (FREDGA et al., 1976) as well as its H-Y antigen expressivity (WACHTEL et al., 1976 b). In view of the established homology of X-linked genes among all mammals (see Table 1), it would appear that the genome of every mammalian species is endowed with this X-linked locus, its wild-type allele being essential for the expression of H-Y antigen.

No one would argue that Y-autosome as well as Y-X translocations have not caused the development of XX males in a variety of mammalian species. However, to regard these translocations as the sole cause of testicular organization, and therefore of H-Y antigen expression in the apparent absence of the Y, is about as unrealistic as regarding sex chromosome mosaicism as the one and only cause of true hermaphrodism. One or more autosomal gene loci appear to be genuinely involved in the expression of H-Y antigen, not including autosomal genes for β_2-microglobulin and MHC antigens. For example, Cattanach found no evidence indicating the Y-chromosome origin of his autosomal dominant Sxr gene of the mouse (CATTANACH et al., 1971). In the goat, XX males and true hermaphrodites are caused by an autosomal, not dominant but recessive gene, either very closely linked to or identical with the mutant gene responsible for the polled (hornless) condition, which incidentally is a dominant trait (HAMERTON et al., 1969).

As far as I know HAMERTON (1968) was the first to give serious consideration to the apparent involvement of non-Y-linked genes in the mammalian primary (gonadal) sex-determining mechanism. Since these non-Y-linked genes have subsequently been shown to be involved in H-Y antigen expression, the testis-determining gene product that Hamerton hypothesized can now be identified as H-Y antigen. Viewed in this light, his conclusion can be stated as follows: The H-Y structural gene resides on the X chromosome while the Y chromosome carries its activator gene. XX males, with an autosomal testis-determining mechanism, might simply have developed an autosomal mimic of this switching action normally carried out by the Y-linked gene.

Regardless of where the H-Y structural gene resides, the involvement of two or more genes in the expression of H-Y antigen, which is constitutive as well as ubiquitous, and which can neither be induced nor be suppressed by hormonal agents, appears redundant and superfluous. Only when one realizes that the H-Y antigen started as one of the inducible gene products in the gonadal development of lower vertebrates, the pivotal role it plays in the primary sex-determining meachanism of mammals being a recent evolutionary acquisition, can we understand the apparently redundant and superfluous involvement of more than one gene in H-Y antigen expression.

a) Flexibility in Gonadal Development of Lower Vertebrates

Despite the extreme evolutionary conservation and its invariably heterogametic-sex-specific appearance (WACHTEL et al., 1975 a), H-Y antigen does not appear to play as pivotal a role in lower vertebrates as it does in the mammalian sex-determining mechanism. In the Japanese cyprinodont fish, Oryzias latipes, the XX/XY scheme of the sex-determining meachanism based on the male heterogamety again operates. Furthermore, because of a close linkage between the sex-determining locus and one of the body color loci, X^rX^r white females and X^rY^R ruby-colored males can be distinguished at a glance. In this species, however, the larval exposure to androgenic and estrogenic steroids readily causes functional sex reversals, producing X^rX^r white males and X^rY^R ruby-colored females, both of which are fertile. By mating ordinary males and sex-reversed females, both of the X^rY^R constitution, Y^RY^R males can be obtained. When they are mated to ordinary X^rX^r females, an all male progeny consisting entirely of ruby-colored X^rY^R fish can be obtained (YAMAMOTO, 1961).

These experiments have shown that sex steroids cause functional sex reversals without altering the genetic sex chromosome constitution. Similarly, in the African clawed toad, Xenopus laevis, the mating between ZW females and sex-reversed ZW males produced WW females, which can also be sex reversed to become functional males (MIKAMO and WITSCHI, 1964). In the chicken and pheasant, it has long been known that either the intentional surgical removal or accidental destruction (e.g., by shotgun pellets) of the left functional ovary of ZW hens often initiates the testicular transformation of the right residual gonad, thus producing a cock with spermatogenesis, although sterile for a simple anatomical reason (BENOIT, 1923; MILLER, 1938). It should be recalled that despite such flexibility in the development of their gonads, the H-Y antigen has been found in the heterogametic ZW female but not in the male of Xenopus laevis as well as in avian species (WACHTEL et al., 1975 a). Nevertheless, it would appear that in fish, amphibians, and birds, members of both sexes retain the potential to express H-Y antigen. Furthermore, the normal expression of this antigen by the heterogametic sex can be suppressed, whereas the same antigen in the homogametic sex can be induced by sex steroid hormones and other means. As shall be discussed in Part III, the expression of the same structural gene can be constitutive in one cell type, while being inducible by a steroid hormone in another. The study of H-Y antigen on sex-reversed ZW testis and ZZ ovary of Xenopus laevis, for example, will be of extreme interest.

A structural gene that can be induced as well as suppressed is obviously under the control of a number of other genes. The persistent involvement of a number of genes in the constitutive and ubiquitous expression of mammalian H-Y antigen can be viewed as an evolutionary relic. Mammalian embryos of both sexes develop in a maternal environment dominated by female sex steroids. The testis-organizing H-Y of mammalian male embryos had to escape from the suppressive control by a female sex steroid to become constitutive in its expression and, by so doing, began to play a pivotal role in the primary sex-determining mechanism. Of the minimum of three genes, one Y-linked, the other X-linked, and the third autosomal involved in the H-Y antigen expression, one has to represent the H-Y structural gene. We shall now consider merits and short-comings of various alternatives.

b) What If the H-Y Structural Gene Is Y-Linked?

The Y linkage of the H-Y structural gene is, of course, the simplest and most straightforward of all the alternatives. The evidence in its favor is the finding that the H-Y antigen level of human XYY males is noticeably higher (200%?) than that of normal XY males (WACHTEL et al., 1975c). However, if this is taken to mean the clear gene dosage effect shown by the Y-linked H-Y structural gene, a problem arises in that we can no longer assign any H-Y antigen-related function to either the X-linked gene or an autosomal one, although each of them is known to be involved in H-Y antigen expression. The manifestation of clear gene dosage effect in its activity by a structural gene reveals that it is not under stringent control of a regulatory gene. If that is the case, how does an X-linked mutation manage to produce fertile XY wood lemming females by suppressing the normal Y chromosome from expressing its H-Y structural gene?

On the other hand, our study of H-Y antigen levels of human male Burkitt lymphoma lines indicated the modulation by a regutatory system of H-Y structural gene activity, for tetraploidization did not result in the doubling of H-Y antigen sites per cell (BEUTLER et al., 1978). The H-Y antibody absorption capacity remained the same between Raji and Tetra Raji (Table 3), and this was also true of another diploid-tetraploid pair, Daudi and Daudi x Daudi self-hybrid. In the above study, overly suppressive modulation of H-Y antigen levels by the tetraploid nucleus was clearly evident.

The concept of the one and only H-Y structural gene residing in the Y chromosome encounters further difficulties in explaining various abnormal situations of testicular organization in the apparent absence of the Y. If each autosomal gene, independently capable of testicular organization, invariably represents the Y-originated H-Y structural gene, why is it that such an autosomal gene behaves as a dominant in the mouse (CATTANACH et al., 1971) and man (KASDAN et al., 1973), whereas it behaves as a recessive in the goat (HAMERTON et al., 1969)?

If one wants to insist on the Y-linkage of the H-Y structural gene, the only way out of the above-noted difficulties can be found in the concept of multiple gene copies in tandem repeats. The grossly heteromorphic XY sex chromosome pair of mammals must have evolved from the homomorphic and essentially homologous XY pair commonly found among fish and amphibians. This evolutionary differentiation has been accomplished exclusively at the expense of the Y chromosome, which underwent genetic degeneration to become a specialized testis determiner, while the X chromosome remained invariant (see Table I). It has been argued that as a result of this specialization, the mammalian Y chromosome came to contain the testis-determining gene in multiple copies (OHNO 1967).

Genes in multiple copies, such as those for 18S and 28S *ribosomal* RNAs residing in the nucleolar-organizing region of a chromosome, show peculiar characteristics of their own. Their transcriptional activities in different cell types are regulated at various levels that seldom exceed 50% of the maximum capacity (CUTLER, 1973/1974). This allows a wide fluctuation in the number of gene copies among healthy individuals of a population, a deleterous effect manifesting itself only when a copy number falls below the critical lower threshold (RITTOSA et al., 1966). On certain occasions, gene copies detach themselves from a chromosome in the episome-like form (BROWN and DAWID, 1968). Apparently for this reason, a group of gene copies can be inserted into a nonhomologous chromosome without the benefit of *bona fide* translocations, i.e., in addition to the known nucleolar-organizing regions, small clusters of ribosomal RNA genes may be found on other nonhomologous chromosomes (PARDUE and HSU, 1975). If the Y-linked testis-organizing H-Y structural genes exist in multiple copies, its activity will be modulated by a regulatory gene residing on the X chromosome. Depending upon whether or not the number of gene copies transferred to an autosome falls below the critical lower threshold of modulatability by a regulatory gene, a newly arisen autosomal festis-organizer can behave either as a recessive or as a dominant. Furthermore, a *bona fide* translocation involving chromosome breaks and reunions is no longer *conditio sine qua non* of a transfer of gene copies from the Y to an autosome. Lower than normal levels of H-Y antigen, so often encountered on human XX males and true hermaphrodites, can readily be explained by the number of H-Y gene copies transferred to an autosome or to the X being insufficient to allow the normal male level H-Y antigen expression by modulation. Similarly, subnormal H-Y antigen levels seen in XY women with pure gonadal dysgenesis can also be explained by a substantial loss of H-Y gene copies from their Y chromosome. Needless to say, the X-linked regulatory gene that modulates H-Y antigen levels can also mutate to become overly repressive. Such a mutation explains the development of fertile XY wood lemming females (FREDGA et al.,1976).

It should be recalled that an autosomal dominant Sxr gene of the mouse is capable of H-Y antigen expression, and therefore of testicular organization in the absence of the Y. Keeping in mind the possible Y-linkage of the H-Y structural gene in multiple copies, S. S. Wachtel and I carefully compared H-Y antigen levels of the three kinds of males of our Sxr stock. They were: (1) carrier XY, Sxr/- males, (2) noncarrier XY, -/- males, and (3) sex-reversed, sterile XX, Sxr/- males with Sertoli-cell-only seminiferous tubules (Fig. 19, left). As schematically illustrated in Fig. 23, the following three hypotheses as to the normal location and number of genes lead to distinctly different predictions as to expected H-Y antigen levels of the three types of males of our Sxr stock: (1) the Y-linkage of the one and only structural gene for H-Y antigen (horizontal column A), (2) an autosomal inheritance of the one and only H-Y structural gene, the Y chromosome carrying its activator gene (horizontal column B), and (3) the Y-linkage of the H-Y structural gene in multiple copies, the X chromosome carrying its modulator gene (horizontal column C).

According to the first hypothesis, carrier XY, Sxr/- males are the functional equivalent of XYY males. Consequently, their H-Y antigen level is expected to be as high as that of XYY males; 200% of that shown by noncarrier XY, -/- males. An autosomal dominant Sxr of the second hypothesis represents a constitutively mutated H-Y structural gene that no longer requires the Y-linked activating gene for its expression. Accordingly, the H-Y antigen level of sex-reversed XX, Sxr/- males reflects the constitutive H-Y antigen level by a single dose of Sxr gene. Because this level was determined to be 80% of that of noncarrier XY, -/- males, XY, Sxr/- males were expected to show a H-Y antigen level of 130%. The actual result was that no difference was found in the H-Y antigen level between carrier XY, Sxr/- males and noncarrier XY, -/- males. This level, in turn, was no different from that of normal XY males of other mouse strains, e.g., BALB/c, C57B/6. The level shown by sex-reversed XX, Sxr/- males was slightly less, roughly 80%, as already noted. Within the range covered by the three types of males of our Sxr stock, the gene dosage effect was not all obvious: Their H-Y antigen levels were very well modulated indeed. The third hypothesis, which implies the Y-linkage of the H-Y structural gene in mulitple copies, emerged as the most plausible of the three alternatives shown in Fig. 23. At the moment, this hypothesis can explain all the abnormal and exceptional variations in gonadal developments encountered in various mammalian species.

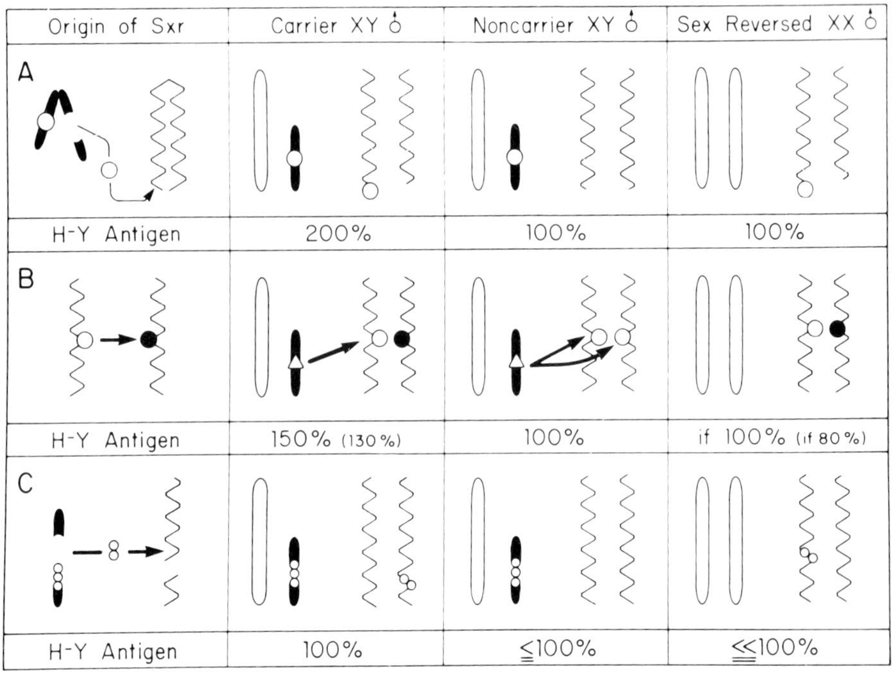

Fig. 23 A-C. Schematic illustration of the three alternatives for the site and numbers of the H-Y structural gene and the resulting different predictions on H-Y antigen levels of the three types of male mice found in our mouse stock in which an autosomal dominant Sxr gene is maintained. The three types of males are: (1) Carrier XY, Sxr/- fertile male, (2) noncarrier XY, -/- fertile male, and (3) sex-reversed XX, Sxr/- sterile male. The fourth alternative, based on the X-linkage of the H-Y structural gene, being controlled by the Y-linked activator and an autosomal repressor, is discussed in the text. It is not included here, for it offers a few alternatives instead of one definite prediction. From *left* to *right* of each column, the X-chromosome is represented by a *long outlined rod*, and the Y, by a *short solid black rod*. A pair of autosomes involved in Sxr are drawn as a pair of *wavy lines*. Each testis-determining H-Y structural gene is represented by an *outlined circle*. In Row B, a *solid black circle* denotes a constitutively mutated H-Y gene (Sxr), whereas an *outlined triangle* on the Y Iindicates an activating gene that is required for the expression of H-Y antigen specified by the wild-type structural gene (*outlined circle*) on an autosome. **A** The Y-linked single copy hypothesis. According to this carrier XY males should show twice the H-Y antigen level of noncarrier XY males. **B** The autosomally inherited single copy hypothesis. Unless a constitutive H-Y antigen level shown by sex-reversed XX males is less than 50% of the noncarrier XY male level, carrier XY males should show a higher than normal H-Y antigen level. **C** The Y-linked multiple (5 in the scheme) copy hypothesis: If a split between the Y and an autosome of the gene copies was more or less even, all three types of males should show about the normal male level of H-Y antigen

c) What If the H-Y Structural Gene Is X-Linked ?

There is yet a fourth alternative. As already noted, the germ of the fourth alternative was proposed by HAMERTON (1968). The examples given at the beginning of this chapter indicated that although the expression of H-Y antigen is also heterogametic-sex-specific in fish and amphibians, the hormonal treatment can induce this antigen in the homogametic sex and cause sex reversals. Conversely, H-Y antigen expression can be repressed by another set of hormonal treatments on the heterogametic sex, causing functional sex reversals in the opposite direction. Obviously, both sexes of gonochoristic fish and amphibians are potentially capable of expressing the H-Y antigen that is testis-organizing in the XX/XY scheme while ovary-organizing in the ZW/ZZ scheme of sex-determining mechanisms.

This effectively precludes the heterogametic-sex-specific Y- as well as W-linkage of the H-Y structural gene. The X- or Z-linkage becomes more attractive. Since H-Y antigen can apparently be induced by steroid hormones and by other means in lower vertebrates, the H-Y activating gene might have resided in the homologous region of the X and the Y as well as of the Z and the W. In mammals, the X-linked H-Y activating gene might have become extinct, thus allowing the constitutive and noninducible H-Y antigen expression only in the heterogametic sex. In lower vertebrates, H-Y antigen expression by the heterogametic sex can apparently be suppressed by steroid hormones and other means. There must have been a H-Y repressing gene, which might have resided on a autosome.

From an evolutionary point of view, the X-linkage of the H-Y structural gene is plausible, the Y-linked activating gene and an autosomal repressing gene controlling its expression. According to this alternative, testicular organization in the absence of the Y is caused either by an autosomal mimic of the Y-linked activator (HAMERTON, 1968), or by a defective mutation of the autosomal repressor. XY females are caused by a defective mutation of either the X-linked H-Y structural gene as in the wood lemming, or by the Y-linked activating gene.

It seems to me that the two remaining viable alternatives, the Y-linkage of the H-Y structural gene in multiple copies and the X-linkage of the H-Y structural gene either in single or multiple copies, are equally attractive. Only if, in the future, it is shown that in certain specific circumstances, H-Y antigen can be induced on normal XX gonadal cells, will the Y-linked hypothesis have to be abandoned in favor of the X-linked one. This brings us to the problem of bovine freemartin gonads.

d) The Origin of H-Y Antigen in Virilized Bovine Freemartin Gonads as an Enigma

The fact that somewhat sexually ambiguous sterile heifers are often born co-twin to bulls must have been known even to prehistoric breeders of cattle. Vascular anastomosis between heterosexual dizygotic twins early in their development was established as the cause of bovine freemartinism by KELLER and TANDLER (1917) as well as by LILLIE (1917) 50 years ago. Naturally, androgenic hormones transferred from a bull fetus *via* anastomosed blood vessels to a genetic female was thought to be the cause of virilization of the latter. As shall be extensively discussed in Part III, we now know that while testosterone is capable of inducing complete extragonadal masculine development in female fetuses, it is totally incapable of altering ovarian organogenesis by mammalian female embryos. In bovine freemartins, it is the gonad that becomes virilized to resemble a minute testis in extreme cases. Often rudimentary development of wolffian duct derivatives has been shown to be caused by androgens synthesized by their own virilized gonads (SHORT et al., 1969). Thus, a twin bull fetus must give something other than androgenic steroids to virilize the XX gonad of a freemartin.

Virilization of the freemartin gonad is very different from testicular organogenesis by normal bull fetuses for it occurs very late in development. The first abnormality noted was the cessation of germ cell multiplication, as well as of organ growth, during gestational days 50 to 60. Definite testicular transformation, if it is to take place, begins only at about the 90th day (JOST et al., 1975). The observation that, when vascular anastomosis between heterosexual dizygotic twins was severed before the 45th day, no virilization of the XX gonad occurred (VIGIER et al., 1976) suggested that testicular transformation of the bovine freemartin gonad requires constant blood-borne stimuli from its bull co-twin.

Choosing extremely virilized small-testis-like gonads of three freemartin fetuses in gestational days 150 to 175, we studied the possible presence of H-Y antigen on these virilized XX gonadal cells. Within the range of cell numbers used for H-Y antibody absorption tests, H-Y antigen was just as prominent in these freemartin gonadal cells as in testicular cells of their bull co-twins (OHNO et al., 1976). Testicular transformation of bovine freemartin gonads, which is a rather rare event, was clearly due to the presence of H-Y antigen. The problem lies in elucidating the origin of this antigen found in XX freemartin gonads.

In 1962, we reported the recovery of XX mitotic figures from newborn testes of two bull calves born co-twins to freemartins. One pair of testes, in fact, yielded twice as many XX mitotic figures as XY Ones. Since somatic elements of the gonad do not migrate, they do not become blood-borne. Accordingly, these XX cells were tentatively identified as donor primordial germ cells that became blood-borne during their migration and found a home in the XX gonad of its co-twin (OHNO et al., 1962). As repeatedly noted, XX primordial germ cells in the testicular environment are incapable of undergoing neonatal differentiation into definitive spermatogonia. It would appear that in our study, we have caught these XX germ cells just before their inevitable extinction. The report of finding heterosexual gonadal chimerisms in freemartin as well as in bull twins continued (KANAGAWA et al., 1965; WEISS and HOFFMANN, 1969), while negative findings have been reported with equal frequency.

In their critical reexamination of the problem, FORD and EVANS (1977) found no XX cells in testes of bull twins, which is no surprise, for these were postnatal samples. However they found three XY mitotic figures among 18 metaphases recovered from the direct preparation of one freemartin gonad. It would appear that the gonadal chimerism in bovine dizygotic twins is a reality. Nevertheless, the presence of XY cells in the midst of XX gonads does not seem to be the cause of gonadal changes so peculiar to bovine freemartins. As discussed extensively in Chap. 8, XX/XY mosaic or chimeric gonads of other mammalian species most often organize functional testes and less often also functional ovaries. Freemartin gonads, in sharp contrast, are essentially dysgenetic. Even when they are virilized enough to resemble a testis in its architecture, its minute size is the most outstanding feature. Furthermore, these donor XY cells in the freemartin gonad do not appear to be the source of H-Y antigen so abundantly present in extremely virilized ones. If they were, the severance of vascular anastomosis between heterosexual twins before the 45th day should not have stopped virilization of the freemartin gonad.

It is of interest here to mention the contrasting situation found in marmoset monkeys. Dizygotic twinning and vascular anastomosis between the twins are the rule of pregnancy in marmoset monkeys. Yet, heterosexual twinning does not affect the fertility of females in the slightest, despite the fact that gonadal chimerism has also been reported in testes as well as in ovaries of these marmoset twins (BENIRSCHKE and BROWNHILL, 1963; HAMPTON, 1970).

We therefore concluded that, in determining the developmental fate of gonads, somatic elements originating from the central gonadal blastema of an emerging gonadal ridge (GROPP and OHNO, 1966) play a far more decisive role than migrant germ cells. Inasmuch as only primordial germ cells are involved in gonadal chimerisms associated with heterosexual twinnings of cattle as well as marmoset monkeys, donor germ cells are incapable of altering the developmental fate of the host gonad. The developmental strategy of competitive displacements, discussed extensively in Chap. 8, must mainly involve somatic elements when applied to the fate of gonads.

The cause of bovine freemartinism and, therefore, the source of H-Y antigen found in extremely virilized freemartin gonads should be sought elsewhere. There must be something very peculiar in male fetal development of the family, *Bovidae*. Jost seems to express the opinion that initial suppression of gonadal growth as well as the regression of müllerian ducts observed in freemartin fetuses is caused by the blood-borne antimüllerian hormone (formerly known as factor X) derived from testicular Sertoli cells of their bull twins (JOST et al., 1977). Such a massive dissemination of the antimüllerian hormone into the blood stream by male fetuses, if proved true, must be one of the peculiarities of *Bovidae*. Lateral true hermaphrodites of most mammalian species, including man, demonstrate the regression of müllerian duct and the development of wolffian duct derivatives only on the side of the testis, while having the developed müllerian duct derivatives on the side of the ovary (OVERZIER, 1963).

This finding clearly reveals that since the amount of antimüllerian hormone normally secreted by a fetal testis is barely enough to have a local effect in the vicinity of that testis, a blood-borne influence is out of the question. The very existence of lateral true hermaphrodites also reveals that the amount of H-Y antigen disseminated by a testis as a testis-organizing hormone is also too small to exert a blood-borne effect. It may be that cattle are peculiar in this respect as well, and that a massive amount of H-Y antigen disseminated into the blood stream by the bull twin's testes is responsible for the virilization of the freemartin gonad. Conversely, the antimüllerian hormone derived from a bull twin may trigger the production of H-Y antigen by XX gonadal cells of the freemartin gonad. If the future proves the potential of XX gonadal cells to synthesize their own H-Y antigen if properly stimulated, the H-Y structural gene clearly does not reside on the Y chromosome either in a single or in multiple copies. The X-linkage of the H-Y structural gene becomes most likely.

A massive dissemination into the blood stream of antimüllerian hormone, as well as testis-organizing H-Y antigen by fetal bull testes, hypothesized above as a peculiarity of cattle, should bring about predictable consequences. In lateral true hermaphrodites, a high circulating concentration of antimüllerian hormone should cause the total regression of müllerian ducts on both sides. This, then, is the expected phenotype of lateral true hermaphrodites peculiar to cattle predicted by Jost. A high circulating concentration of testis-organizing H-Y antigen, on the other hand, should not permit the development of lateral true hermaphrodites in cattle. The absence of this particular type of true hermaphrodites then becomes the predicted consequence.

Part III

Nuclear-Cytosol Androgen-Receptor Protein and Hormonal Secondary (Extragonadal) Sex Determination

Chapter 11

The Inherently Feminine Embryonic Plan and Testosterone Induction of the Male Secondary Sex

In Part II, we saw that the primary (gonadal) sex of mammals is indeed determined by a genuine genetic difference between the sexes. The constitutive production of testis-organizing H-Y antigen by male embryos diverted the embryonic gonad's inherent tendency to develop into an ovary and caused the testicular organization. Although the constitutive expression of H-Y antigen is, as a rule, associated with the male-specific occurrence of the Y chromosome, in exceptional species and individuals we have seen that in a very strict sense, it is the expression or nonexpression of H-Y antigen rather than the presence or absence of the Y that determines the fate of embryonic gonads. With the successful organization of testes, the task assigned to the male-specific gene, has been accomplished regardless of whether it represents the H-Y structural gene or its regulator. Although the Y chromosome may perform a few other tasks, such as preventing the manifestation of the webbed neck and exceptionally short stature in the absence of the second X in man or ensuring the motility of spermatozoa in the mouse, such peripheral problems do not belong to the realm covered by this book.

Provided that none of the genes belonging to the regulatory hierarchy activated by H-Y antigen has sustained a deleterious mutation, the H-Y antigen-organized embryonic testis soon begins its assigned endocrine functions. Its Leydig cells start active synthesis and secretion of testosterone and its Sertoli cells the anti-müllerian hormone. The ability of these testicular cells to synthesize the above two hormones does not depend upon the male-specific gene, for Chapter 8 has shown that genetically female XX gonadal cells, when their plasma membranes are endowed with H-Y antigen, differentiate into functional Leydig and Sertoli cells. Furthermore, males and females, and therefore testes and ovaries, utilize the same set of enzymes for their sex steroid hormone synthesis. Thus, one of the female hormones, progesterone, is a precursor of androstenedione, which is an immediate precursor of testosterone. The microsomal aromatase, present in various cell types of both sexes, is responsible for the conversion of androstenedione to estrone, which is an immediate precursor of the second female hormone, estradiol-17β. Male and female steroid hormones are indeed the products of the same synthetic pathway. Therefore, it is no surprise to find that, when circulating testosterone of immunized female rabbits was rendered ineffective by its specific antibody, their testosterone level approached that of normal adult males. The negative feedback gonadotropin secretion inhibition mechanism of the hypothalamo-pituitary axis is apparently incapable of sensing antibody-bound testosterone (BIDLINGMAIER et al., 1977).

To be sure, there is a distinct sexual difference in the gonadotropin regulation of sex steroid synthesis. This too, however, is no reflection of an intrinsic difference between genetically male and female extragonadal cells. This sex difference is simply created by the occurrence or nonoccurrence of the neonatal imprinting of the hypothalamo-pituitary axis by sex steroids.

It is a curious fact that man through the ages appears to have been fascinated by the idea of finding a creature who is made of the right half of a man and the left half of a woman fused into one. In medieval drawings and paintings, such a creature was called an androgyny. Although, as already noted, there are lateral true hermaphrodites with an ovary and müllerian duct derivatives on one side, and a testis and wolffian duct derivatives on the other, such a vertical midline split is confined strictly to the inner organs. There is no left-right asymmetry in their external sexual development. Their circulating testosterone levels uniformly determine the extent of masculine manifestations e.g., beard growth, penis size, etc. while their circulating estradiol levels control the extent of postpubertal feminine manifestation, e.g., breast fullness, hip roundness, etc., their XX and XY cells are equally responsive to testosterone as well as to estradiol. Thus, the androgyny, as a figment of unrealistic imagination, most effectively illustrates the total hormonal dependence of the mammalian secondary sex-determining mechanism. Androgynies, here known as gynandromorphs, do occur among those insects in which the sex-determining mechanism operates based on the XO/XX scheme of male heterogamety. A nondisjunctional event occurring in an early cleavage division of the XX zygote produces an XX/XO mosaic. One-half of the body, populated by XX cells, manifests the feminine phenotype whereas the other half, populated by X0 cells, assumes the appearance of a male. In insects, the extragonadal sex is also determined by the intrinsic property of individual cells. It should be recalled that in mammals, XY/XX mosaics and chimeras most often develop as normal males.

a) Testosterone and Fetal Development of Secondary Sex

At the time of embryonic development when the fate of the gonads is about to be determined, mammalian embryos of both sexes are equipped with a pair of parallely running ducts on each side, which open into the cloaca: the wolffian (mesonephric) duct system and the müllerian (paramesonephric) duct system. Subsequent development of müllerian ducts to fallopian tubes, the uterus and vagina, and of the urogenital sinus and external genitalia to vaginal vestibule, clitoris, labia minora and majora, is an intrinsically programmed developmental process that requires no inducer. The complete regression of wolffian ducts is also an intrinsic process whose prevention requires active intervention. Indeed, the basic mammalian embryonic plan is inherently feminine with regard to the secondary sex determination as well. Accordingly, male embryos castrated at a properly early stage follow the above-noted intrinsic developmental pathway and acquire feminine secondary sex chracteristics (JOST, 1947a). Imediately following the castration of male embryos, if they are continuously exposed to exogenously supplied testosterone by daily treatments of their mother, not only these castrated males, but also their sisters acquire the male secondary sex chracteristics. Wolffian ducts develop into epididymis, ductus deferens, seminal vesicles, and ejaculatory ducts, while the urogenital sinus and external genitalia are masculinized to form the prostate, scrotum, and penis (JOST, 1947b). In this manner, the survival and differentiation of wolffian ducts, and the masculinization of the urogenital sinus and external genitalia, have been established as an entirely androgen-dependent developmental process.

This tetosterone treatment, however, does not cause the regression of müllerian ducts either in castrated males or intact females. Obviously, the fetal testis secretes another factor, which has the singular function of causing regression of müllerian ducts. This factor has now been identified as the anti müllerian hormone, which is thought to be a large peptide synthesized by testicular Sertoli cells (JOSSO et al., 1977). The process of fetal secondary sex determination is schematically summarized in Fig. 24.

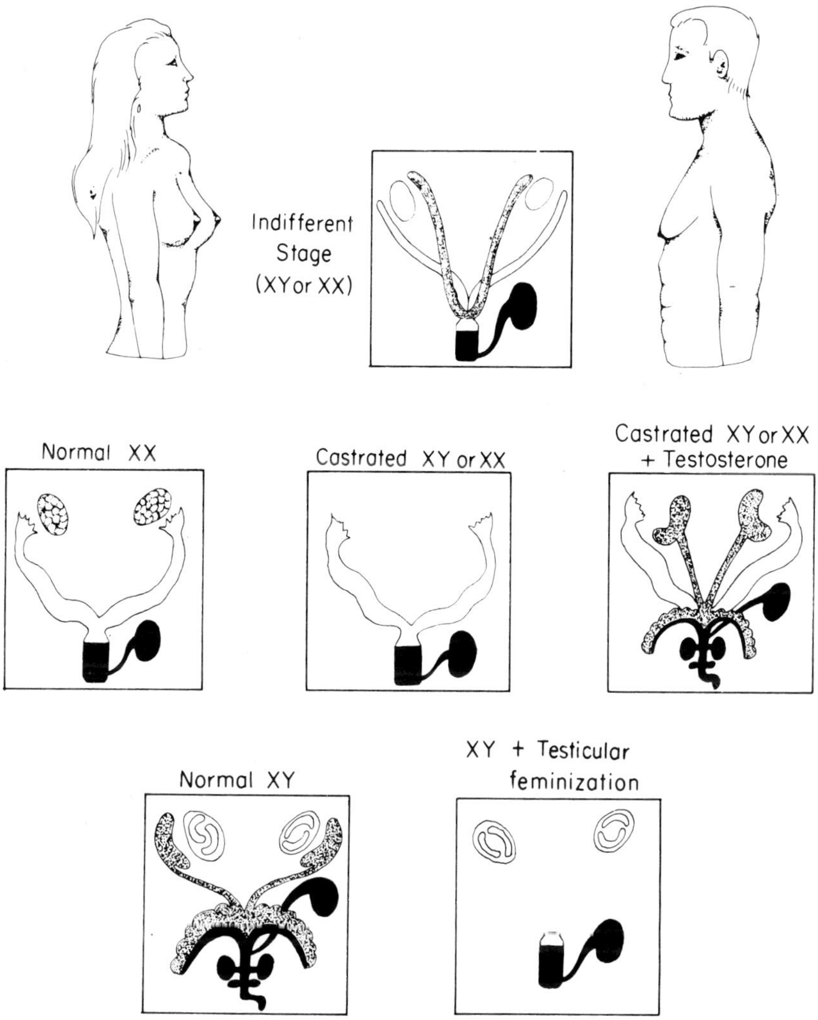

Fig. 24. A scheme showing the testosterone dependence of the mammalian secondary sex-determining mechanism on the fate of wolffian ducts (*shaded*), müllerian ducts (*outlined*) and urogenital sinus (*solid black*). The pair of beanshaped bodies at the top of each square signify gonads: indifferent gonaf (*outlined*), ovary (*filled with small circles*), and testes (*containing two tubules*)

In rodents, but not in man, testosterone-induced masculine differentiation includes the severance of the connection between the nipple and underlying mammary glands. As a result, male nipples become far less conspicuous than female ones (RAYNAUD, 1947). Also in rodents, secondary sex determination involves a sexual differentiation of the central nervous system at the neonatal stage. Within a few days after birth, circulating testosterone of male neonates, either directly or indirectly, imprints masculine charateristics on the hypothalamic region. Because this process constitutes the last in a series of testosterone-induced extragonadal masculine developmental steps, the experimental imprinting of female neonates can easily be done by a single administration of testosterone. In this manner, it was found that the masculinized hypothalamo-pituitary axis is incapable of manifesting the positive feedback response to a rising level of circulating estradiol, which, in nonimprinted females, should have caused a massive release of LH (luteinizing hormone) to induce ovulations to complete the estrous cycle. Accordingly, females with the neonatally masculinized central nervous system exhibit the so-called constant estrus syndrome (HARRIS, 1964). These neonatally masculinized females, if properly primed postpubertally, also manifest masculine sexual behavior: attacking adult males and attempting to mount estrous females. In addition, the neonatal imprinting of the hypothalamo-pituitary axis appears to alter the pattern of hepatic steroid metabolism (GUSTAFSSON and STEINBERG, 1976). As to man, when all the available evidence is weighed, masculine imprinting of the central nervous system does not appear to constitute an integral part of the secondary sex-determining mechanism (MONEY, 1965).

The neonatal masculinization of the central nervous system, as well as the postpubertal elicitation and maintenance of masculine sexual behavior, however, are emerging as constituents of a unique paradox with an element of poetic justice, for it now appears that it is not testosterone *per se* but a female hormone, estradiol-17β, converted *in situ* from testosterone, which is responsible for the manifestation of the above-noted portions of the oft-exulted masculinity. It has been known for some time that a smaller dose of estradiol is as effective as testosterone in masculinizing the hypothalamic region of neonates (GORSKI, 1966), and that the specific neurons in the septal-preoptic-hypothalamic axis, amygdala and hippocampus, retain estradiol more efficiently than testosterone (PFAFF, 1971). More recently, the hypothalamic region has been shown to contain an abundance of microsomal aromatase, which is obviously responsible for the *in situ* conversion of testosterone to estradiol-17β (RYAN et al., 1972). Even the maintenance of postpubertal masculine behavior appears to be the task of *in situ* generated estradiol, for the administration of estradiol instead of testosterone restored masculine behavior to castrated red deer stags (FLECHER and SHORT 1974). It should be pointed out here that while the microsomal aromatase readily converts androstenedione to estrone and testosterone to estradiol, there is no known enzymatic system that can catalyze the reverse conversion of estradiol to testosterone.

In mice, the central nervous system of female neonates is apparently protected from inadvertent masculine imprinting by their own estradiol by a circulating α-fetoprotein, which shows an extremely high binding affinity to this female steroid hormone, thus very effectively reducing the plasma free estradiol concentration available to its target cells (MCEWAN et al., 1975.; ATTARDI and ROUSLAHTI, 1976). Human α-fetoprotein, in sharp contrast, shows no particular binding affinity to estradiol, but then masculine imprinting of the central nervous system does not appear to constitute an integral part of the secondary sex-determining mechanism in man.

b) Fetal Synthesis of Testosterone and the Two Means of Its Delivery to Targets

Inasmuch as the mammalian embryonic plan is inherently feminine, the fetal ovary, having no immediate endocrine function to perform, grows and differentiates at a leisurely pace (Chapter 6). On the contrary, in order to prevent the regression of wolffian ducts by inducing their masculine differentiation, the fetal testis has to function as an endocrine organ almost immediately following completion of its organogenesis. It has to keep playing this role for a considerable period until the forced regression of müllerian ducts as well as induced masculine development of the urogenital sinus and external genitalia has been completed.

While the extremely short gestation period of laboratory mice and rats hinders the identification of this period of intense endocrine activity by the fetal testis, such a period is readily definable in larger mammalian species with long gestation periods, such as man. The newly emerged human testis of gestational day 56 already contains over 4 ng testosterone/mg tissue, the intra testicular testosterone concentration reaching a peak of 5 ng at day 84. The circulating testosterone level reaches its peak of 3.0 ng/ml at about day 112, returning to the charateristically low level of less than 0.5 ng/ml roughly on day 168 (REYES et al., 1974). Indeed, for a period of nearly two months, starting from day 84, circulating testosterone levels of male fetuses approach the low normal testosterone level of adult human males. It is no coincidence that this period of nearly two months corresponds to that during which the urogenital sinus and external genitalia remain amenable to testosterone-induced masculine differentiation. On the other hand, the androgen-sensitive period of wolffian ducts, during which testosterone can prevent their regression by inducing masculine differentiation is considerably shorter and occurs earlier and coincides with a peak in intratesticular testosterone concentration on day 84. In 1971, we proposed that the masculine development of wolffian ducts of male fetuses is not due to circulating testosterone but rather exclusively to testosterone secreted directly from the adjacent testis into the lumen and the immediate surroundings of the wolffian duct (OHNO et al., 1971). As noted at the end of Chap. 10, human lateral true hermaphrodites characteristically demonstrate wolffian duct development on the side of a testis and müllerian duct development on the side of an ovary. It would appear that antimüllerian hormone by a fetal testis is also given by this direct route to each branch fo the müllerian ducts.

This direct route explains the possession of masculinized wolffian duct derivatives by many of the male pseudohermaphrodites having feminine external genitalia. Their defective fetal testes, caused by mutational deficiencies of either androgen-synthesizing enzymes or Leydig cell differentiation, were able to provide a high enough concentration of testosterone to wolffian ducts *via* the direct route but unable to raise the circulating testosterone level high enough to masculinize the urogenital sinus and external genitalia. This was certainly true of a human male pseudohermaphrodite who postpubertally demonstrated a complete Leydig cell agenesis (BERTHEZENE et al., 1976). It is probable that even during normal masculine differentiation, the urogenital sinus and external genitalia have to make do with a lesser concentration of testosterone than the wolffian ducts. A prominent rise in 5α-reductase activity of the urogenital sinus and external genitalia of human fetuses seen before they became amenable to testosterone-induced masculine differentiation (SIITERI and WILSON, 1974) can be viewed as an ontogenetic attempt to compensate for the paucity of available testosterone. The nuclear-cytosol androgen-receptor protein of testosterone target cells certainly demonstrates a higher binding affinity to 5α-dihydrotestosterone than to testosterone itself, as shall be discussed in the next chapter.

The role that the fetal pituitary plays in initiating testosterone synthesis by newly organized testes has long been debated. Nevertheless, more recent evidence apparently favors the view that fetal Leydig cell activity is triggered by chorionic gonadotropin, at least in man. In man, maternal chorionic gonadotropin levels, and therefore fetal levels as well, peak at gestational day 56 to 70 (MARSHALL et al., 1968). In the mouse, an autosomal recessive hpg (hypogonadic) gene, which causes a deficiency of hypothalamic gonadotropic-releasing hormone (GnRH), has been identified (CATTANACH et al., 1977). In the nearly total absence of circulating gonadotropins (FSH as well as LH), homozygotes of both sexes continue to remain sexually infantile; therefore, they are sterile. Nevertheless, hpg/hpg homozygous males are endowed with a complete set of masculine reproductive ducts and accessory organs, thus revealing that their fetal Leydig cells have synthesized enough testosterone to cause the complete masculine differentiation of the wolffian ducts, urogenital sinus, and external genitalia. This seems to reveal rather conclusively that the fetal hypothalamo-pituitary axis is of trivial significance in triggering and maintaining the testosterone synthetic activity of fetal Leydig cells.

In concluding this section, I might impart our own experience with these hpg/hpg adult males. In the untreated state, their reproductive ducts and organs were miniscule in size, but after daily treatment with testosterone as well as with 5α-dihydrotestosterone, these organs and ducts grew to the normal male size.

c) Fetal Versus Postpubertal Response to Testosterone and Mesenchymal Versus Epithelial Cells as Testosterone Targets

The role that testosterone plays in mammalian fetuses is to induce the creation of male-specific, but extragonadal, reproductive organs by promoting the growth and differentiation of wolffian ducts, urogenital sinus, and external genitalia. In this sense, fetal testosterone is involved in organogenesis, the principles of which have been thoroughly discussed in Part II in connection with H-Y antigen-directed testicular oranogenesis. One of the tasks that testosterone performs in this regard is likely to be the induction of a set of cell type-specific plasma membrane antigens; for example, an epididymis-specific plasma membrane antigen to cells comprising a proximal portion of the wolffian duct, and a seminal vesicle-specific plasma membrane antigens to cells of a distal portion of the wolffian duct and/or of a proximal portion of the urogenital sinus.

In addition, however, I feel that testosterone at this stage works mainly through mesenchymal cells to regulate mitotic activities of epithelial cells lying above them. For example, the simple ductal structure of Wolff at its distal end can be induced to branch out glandular structures of the seminal vesicle by locally manipulating the mitotic activity of epithelial elements *via* underlying mesenchymal cells, as schematically illustrated in Fig. 25 in the crudest form. The important role that the underlying mesenchyme plays in organogenesis has long been emphasized by GROBSTEIN (1967). H-Y antigen-directed testicular organization appears to be no exception as discussed in Chapter 7 and illustrated in Fig. 15. With regard to testosterone-dependent masculine differentiation of the urogenital sinus, CUNHA (1972) showed in the mouse that the fetal heterotypic recombinant, made of 12th-day snout dermis mesenchyme and 15th day urogenital sinus epithelium, when grown in the anterior eye chamber of adult males, produces epithelial keratinization, suggesting that, in the absence of androgen-responsive mesenchyme, the urogenital sinus epithelium differentiates as an ordinary epidermis. In sharp contrast, the recombinant composed of 16th-day seminal vesicle mesenchyme and 12-day snout skin epithelium produces single and branched epithelial tubules, suggesting that the androgen-responsive mesenchyme is able to entice

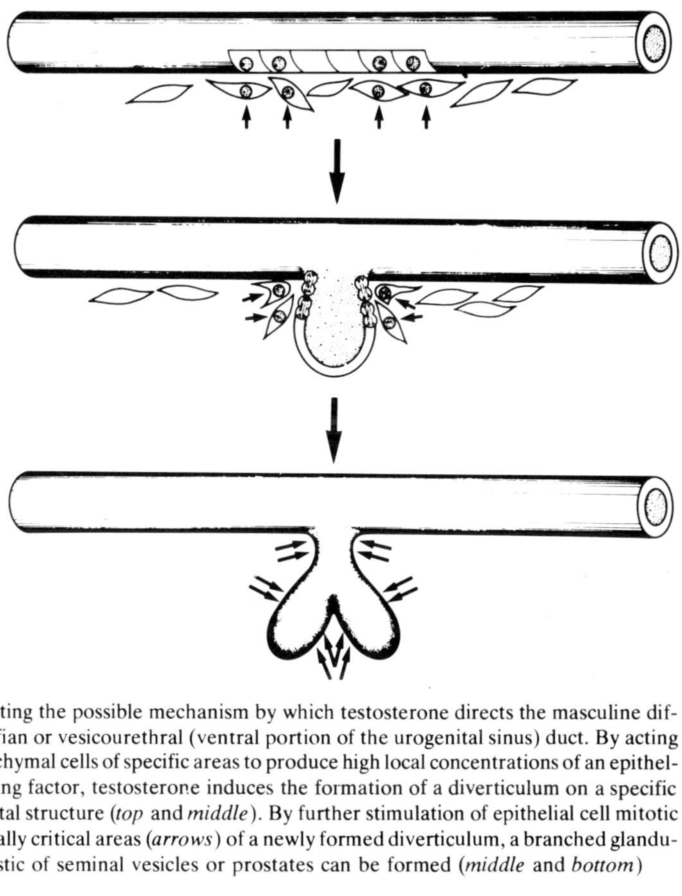

Fig. 25. Scheme illustrating the possible mechanism by which testosterone directs the masculine differentiation of the wolffian or vesicourethral (ventral portion of the urogenital sinus) duct. By acting upon underlying mesenchymal cells of specific areas to produce high local concentrations of an epithelial cell mitosis-stimulating factor, testosterone induces the formation of a diverticulum on a specific position of a simple ductal structure (*top* and *middle*). By further stimulation of epithelial cell mitotic activity at four strategically critical areas (*arrows*) of a newly formed diverticulum, a branched glandular structure characteristic of seminal vesicles or prostates can be formed (*middle* and *bottom*)

ordinary skin epidermal cells to differentiate as though they were seminal vesicle epithelial cells. More shall be said in the next chapter of the androgen dependence of mesenchymal cells.

The role of testosterone in adult males is considerably different. To be sure, male-specific reproductive organs that owe their existence to fetal testosterone undergo further growth triggered by a pubertal rise in circulating testosterone. Such growth due to mitotic activities of epithelial elements is still mediated through underlying mesenchymal fibroblasts.

The evidence in support of this assertion shall be presented in the next chapter. Nevertheless, testosterone now has a new role to perform on these male-specific reproductive organs. By acting directly upon epithelial cells, it induces a specific set of structural gene products in each organ. By so doing, testosterone induces secretory functions in a variety of male accessory glands attached to the reproductive tract. In man, several amines, including noradrenaline, histamine, acetylcholine, and serotonin, have been shown to occur in the tissues comprising the male reproductive tract, often in surprisingly high concentrations. No fewer than 13 prostaglandins have been identified as normal constituents of human seminal plasma. They are thought to contribute to the ejaculatory process by causing contractions of the male reproductive tracts. The prostatic secretions contain citric acid and acid phosphatase in very high concentrations, whereas the vesicular secretion is characterized by a high concentration of fructose (MANN, 1972). Needless to say, epididymis, ductus deferens, seminal vesicles, prostates, penis and scrotum noted above constitute essential reproductive organs of mammalian males. We might call them essential androgen target organs.

In Part I, I noted that a majority of mammals, especially large ones, are sexually dimorphic species that practice polygymous matings. In these sexually dimorphic species, postpubertal testosterone has the task of inducing various symbols of masculine supremacy that are extremely varied and highly species specific. We shall define these additional organs and cell types that become androgen-dependent postpubertally, as symbolic androgen target organs. The testosterone-dependent growth of man's beard, the lion's mane, and the stag's antlers reveal the dominant role that visual cues play in eliciting sexual behavior of these species. The primary function of these symbols appears to be to provoke aggression among adult males rather than to serve as attractants to adult females of the same species, for they often include combative weapons made purposely ineffective. The stag's antlers are an excellent example, as mentioded in Part I. To the extent that victors in male-to-male combat are likely to be endowed with grosser specimens of these symbols, they indirectly serve as attractants to adult females. For the postpubertal growth of these visual symbols of masculine supremacy, testosterone is again likely to work through mesenchymal cells to provide directed mitotic stimuli to the pertinent cell types.

In contrast, symbolic androgen target organs of primarily nocturnal mammalian species are likey to furnish olfactory cues, because as far as this type of target organs is concerned, postpubertal testosterone acts directly upon the epithelial elements to induce specific sets of structural gene products, the consequence of which is the production of pheromones. The case in point is the mouse. Despite its miniscule body size, the male mouse is an extremely aggressive and highly territorial creature. Testosterone induces aggression-provoking body odors in adult males. Thus, if such odors are artificially induced in adult females by a series of testosterone treatments, females now become the object of aggression by adult males (MUGFORD and NOWELL, 1970). Urinary pheromones, with which each adult male continuously marks his own den, enhance his own aggression while retarding that of an intruder. In this way, a decisive combative advantage is given to the resident male when he faces an intruder (JONES and NOWELL, 1974). If two transparent cages, each housing an adult male, are placed immediately adjacent to each other, each male immediately begins a series of urinations along the suddenly created territorial boundary, provided that each male has been reared only with female consorts since the time of puberty, and therefore knows no fear of defeat. Ignorance can indeed be a blessing. Fittingly, submaxillary salivary glands, kidney, and preputial glands, each with excretory functions, have been identified as the symbolic androgen target organs of the mouse. In submaxillary salivary glands, testosterone induces NGF (nerve growth factor) and a few peptidases (LEVI-MONTALCINI and ANGELETTI, 1961). In the kidney, there is a nearly 100-fold induction of alcohol dehydrogenase, which also functions as 3β-hydroxy-5β-steroid dehydrogenase, and of β-glucuronidase, and lesser inductions of esterases and a few other enzymes (DOFUKU et al., 1971a). When kidney sections from androgen-treated mice are histochemically stained for induced β-glucuronidase, epithelial cells of the proximal tubules reveal themselves to be the real target cell types of this symbolic androgen target organ (Fig. 26). Although these target cells become extremely hypertrophic, causing an increase of as much as 45% in wet kidney weight, they do not engage in mitotic activity in response to androgens, thus proving that mesenchymal cells need not be involved in the postpubertal testosterone action.

With regard to direct testosterone action upon epithelial elements, the foregoing discussions disclose the important fact that androgens induce entirely different sets of structural gene products in various target cell types. For example, the mouse genome is endewed with one structural gene each for alcohol dehydrogenase and β-glucuronidase. While both genes are androgen-inducible in the kidney, their expressions are constitutive in the liver: alcohol dehydrogenase at a very high level comparable to the fully induced kidney level, and β-glucuronidase at a very low level barely above the noninduced kidney level. In submaxillary salivary glands, the alcohol dehydrogenase gene is not expressed either in the presence or absence of androgens, while the β-glucuronidase gene is constitutively expressed at the low level and is impervious to the inducing action of androgens (OHNO, 1976c). It is well worth remembering that depending upon the cell type in which it resides, the same structural gene may or may not be included in the regulatory system that utilizes testosterone and its effective metabolite as inducers.

Adult males of the sexually dimorphic species tend to grow considerably larger than adult females. This aspect of postpubertal sexual dimorphism has traditionally been attributed to the so-called anabolic effect of androgens. As far as this particular aspect of testosterone action is concerned, my feeling is that the hypothalamo-pituitary axis serves as a far more important target than skeletal muscle cells. Indeed female mice, with the neonatally masculinized central nervous system acquire the body size and musculature of adult males without the benefit of added postpubertal steroid treatments. Granted, the neonatal masculine imprint-

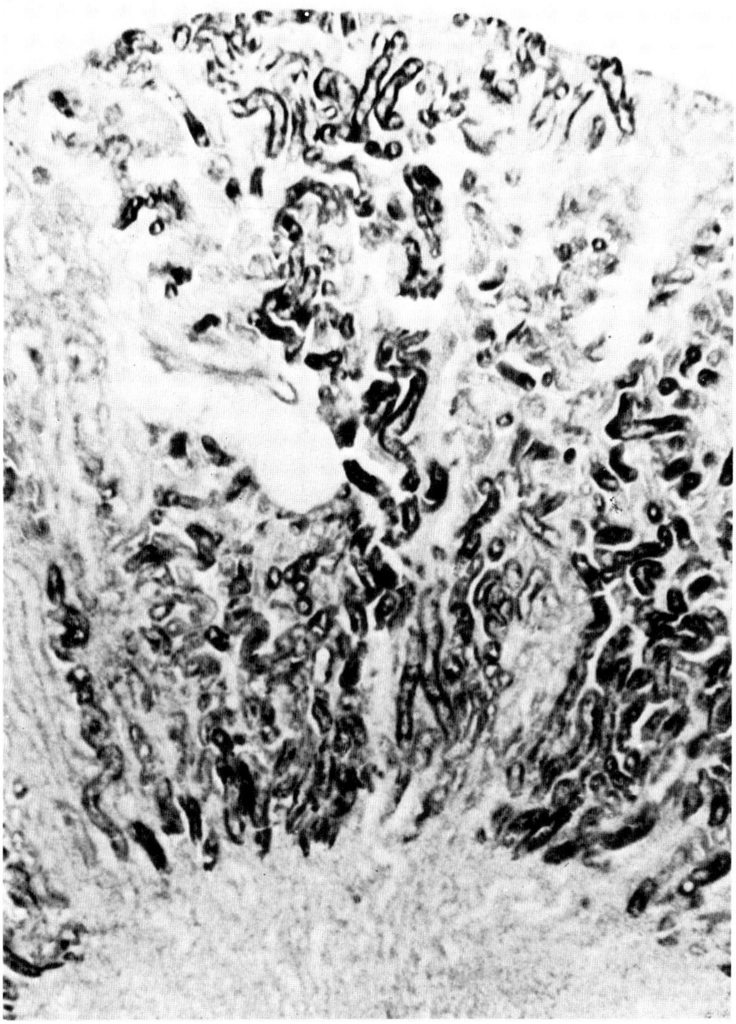

Fig. 26. A photomicrograph of a 5α-dihydrotestosterone-induced female mouse kidney section stained for β-glucuronidase. Only proximal tubule cells in the renal cortex are the real target cell type of androgens. Because this female was heterozygous for an X-linked androgen-insensitive testicular feminization (*Tfm*) mutation, those proximal tubules poulated by Tfm cells are not stained (TETTENBORN, DOFUKU and OHNO, 1971), Lenses used: 2.5 x 10

ing process of the central nervous system may be unique to rodents. Nevertheless, in the larger sexually dimorphic mammalian species also, testosterone at some stage in development may, in a very subtle way, alter the secretory pattern of the pituitary growth hormone and other hormones concerned with the growth of the body as a whole.

d) 5α-Reductase and the Relative Efficacy of Testosterone Versus 5α-Dihydrotestosterone

It has long been recognized that as far as the circulating androgens of mammals are concerned, testosterone is the most effective androgen. However, with the discovery of 5α-reductase in one of the prime androgen target organs, the prostates (BRUCHOVSKY and WILSON, 1968a), a new and exciting thought arose, i.e. that 5α-dihydrotestosterone converted *in situ* from testosterone by the preceding enzyme might actually be the real androgen. Unfortunately, subsequent studies have gradually revealed that not all the androgen target organs are richly endowed with 5α-reductase, and that those poor in 5α-reductase, such as the mouse kidney, tend to metabolize administered 5α-dihydrotestosterone very quickly to 5α-androstandiols (BULLOCK et al., 1971). Consequently the notion of two distinct kinds of androgen target organs began to emerge. According to this notion, those male reproductive organs derived from the urogenital sinus and external genitalia constitute the 5α-dihydrotestosterone target organs, whereas, wolffian duct dericatives and the various symbolic target organs mentioned previously comprise the testosterone target organs. The above notion was made untenable by the observation that the mouse kidney, although incapable of generating an appreciable amount of 5α-dihydrotestosterone of its own by the *in situ* conversion of testosterone, was nevertheless far more responsive to administered 5α-dihydrotestosterone than testosterone (OHNO 1971). Furthermore, the so-called testosterone target organs demonstrated a curious and apparently inexplicable hyperresponsiveness to 5α-androstan-3α-17β-diol, one of the two intratarget metabolites of 5α-dihydrotestosterone. This was true of the adult mouse kidney (OHNO et al., 1971) as well as of the rat embryonic wolffian duct (SCHULTZ and WILSON, 1974).

This phenomenon is no longer inexplicable if my interpretation schematically illustrated in Fig. 27 holds true. Androgen target organs in general are equipped with two sequential steroid-metabolizing enzymes to handle testosterone derived from the circulation. The 5α-dihydrotestosterone target organs are rich in the first enzyme and poor in the second. Accordingly, they retain a significant amount of 5α-dihydrotestosterone. The testosterone target organs, in contrast, are poor in the first but extremely rich in the second enzyme. Thus, in the physiologic fetal as well as postpubertal male environment, they have to make do with testosterone. Nevertheless, their innate preference for 5α-dihydrotestosterone as an inducer is no different from that of the 5α-dihydrotestosterone target organs. While the first inzyme catalyzes the one-way conversion of testosterone to 5α-dihydrotestosterone, the second enzyme catalyzes inter conversions between dihydrotestosterone and androstandiol. I do not believe that this second enzyme is the conventional 3β-hydroxysteroid dehydrogenase (E.C.1.1.1.51), but that it is akin to 3α-hydroxysteroid dehydrogenase (E.C.1.1.1.50), at least in its reverse reaction. Because of the efficacy of the reverse reaction by the second enzyme, the administration of 5α-androstan-3α, 17β-diol causes the so-called testosterone target organs to retain a greater amount of 5α-dihydrotestosterone than the administration of 5α-hydrotestosterone itself; hence, the apparent super efficacy of this androstandiol as an inducer. More shall be said of this androstandiol in the next chapter, when we deal with the nuclear-cytosol androgen-receptor protein.

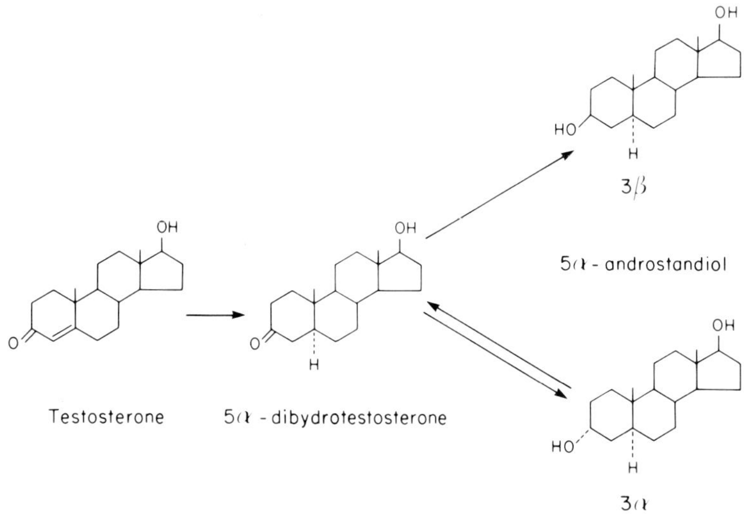

Fig. 27. The metabolism of testosterone within target cells. The first enzyme, 5α-reductase, catalyzes the unidirectional conversion of testosterone to 5α-dihydrotestosterone. The second enzyme in the forward reaction further converts 5α-dihydrotestosterone to two kinds (3α and 3β) of 5α- androstandiol. The so-called 5α-dihydrotestosterone target organs are rich in the first enzyme but poor in the second, whereas the converse is true of the so-called testosterone target organs. Because of the richness in the second enzyme, however, the latter efficiently converts, by the reverse reaction, administered 5α-androstan-3α, 17β-diol to 5α-dihydrotestosterone: hence, an apparent super efficacy of this androstandiol as an inducer of the latter

Regardless of the validity of my hypothesis illustrated in Fig. 27, the fact remains that if we descount a difference in the testosterone-metabolizing capacities noted above, the mammalian body is endowed with only one kind of androgen target organ, all target organs are innately most responsive to 5α-dihydrotestosterone, but, in its absence, testosterone can function as its less efficient substitute. Having to utilize this less efficient substitute as an inducer, the so-called testosterone target organs in the adult male remain only in a partially induced state, 30% of the full capacity in the case of mouse kidney (DOFUKU et al., 1971a), whereas the fully induced state is attained by the 5α-dihydrotestosterone target organs.

Over the millennia, natural selection has adjusted substrate binding affinities of most enzymes in such a way that in the cellular environment, they function at levels considerably below their innate maximal velocities. Such adjustments provided each metabolic pathway with the needed flexibility to deal with constantly changing substrate concentrations. Along the same vein, at the adult male circulating testosterone level of roughly 10^{-8}M, the symbolic androgen target organs of sexually dimorphic males remain in partially induced states. This is of obvious evolutionary significance. The elation following victory in male-to-male combat, and of the subsequent acquisition of additional females to his harem, cause frequent rises in the victor's testosterone level. Thus, he literally grows in stature and his symbols of masculine supremacy become increasingly luxurious, while the vanquished with his reduced testosterone level literally shrinks with shame.

I shall end this chapter with a most enlightening finding reported on one specific form of human male pseudohermaphroditism, locally known as the "guevedoces (penis at 12)" syndrome (IMPERATO - MCGINLEY et al., 1974). At birth, males homozygous for an autosomal recessive 5α-reductase deficiency mutation are equipped with the complete set of wolffian duct derivatives, but their external genitalia are ambiguous enough for them to be raised as girls: labia-like scrotum, a blind vaginal pouch, and clitoris-like phallus. At puberty, however, striking changes take place. Their voices deepen and they develop a typically male physique with a substantial increase in muscle mass, the phallus enlarges to become a functional penis, and an enlarged scrotum now houses the descended testes. In the absence of 5α-reductase, the circulating fetal testosterone level has not been quite sufficient to cause complete masculine development of the urogenital sinus and external genitalia. A higher postpubertal testosterone level, on the other hand, becomes just high enough to remedy most of the initially present deficiencies in the continued absence of 5α-reductase.

Chapter 12

Abolition of All Adrogen Target Organ Responses by the X-Linked Tfm (Testicular Feminization) Mutation

We have seen that both the primary (gonadal) and secondary (extragonadal) sex-determining meachanisms of mammals are founded on the principle of the inherently feminine basic embryonic plan. Accordingly, testis-organizing H-Y antigen has risen to the top of the regulatory hierarchy that determines the fate of embryonic gonads. As soon as fetal Leydig cells of the H-Y antigen-organized testis begin to synthesize and secrete testosterone, the second regulatory hierarchy for extragonadal sexual differentiation is set in motion. If there is to be a master regulatory gene product for the second hierarchical system as well, such a molecule must necessarily mediate the androgen-responsiveness of all the target cell types in the mammalian body. Because no sexual difference in the responsiveness to androgens has been noted either during the critical fetal stage or during the postpubertal stage, the above-noted molecule must be present in males and females alike. Thus, we realize that the two regulatory hierarchies are completely separated from and independent of each other.

Before we proceed with our search for a master regulatory gene product for extragonadal sexual differentiation, however, we must dispense with a minor, but nevertheless totally independent, component of the secondary sex-determination

It should be recalled that in the continuous presence of exogenous androgen, müllerian ducts of both castrated male and intact female fetuses manage to differentiate into fallopian tubes, uterus, and vagina (see Fig. 24). Thus androgen that induces masculine differentiation of wolffian ducts, the urogenital sinus, and external genitalia, is totally incapable of causing the regression of müllerian ducts. As already mentioned on several occasions, this task has been assigned to the antimüllerian peptide hormone secreted by thy fetal Sertoli cells (JOSSO et al., 1977). There is an accessory regulatory system consisting essentially of the two components: the above noted hormone and its specific plasma membrane receptor on cells of the embryonic müllerian duct. The gene locus for one or the other of the above two components can sustain a deleterious mutation and should result in the persistence of müllerian duct derivatives in otherwise normal males. Such a condition has apparently been recognized in human male patients since the nineteenth century. Of various headings under which this condition has been described, the persistens oviduct syndrome appears most appropriate (MORILLO CUCCI and GERMAN, 1971). It seems as though this trait is inherited as an autosomal recessive (LENZ, 1954). Which of the two loci, one for the hormone and the other for its specific receptor, is involved in the above defect cannot be known until the study on affected fetuses of an appropriate state is made.

Now that that an accessory regulatory system has been dealt with, we can return to the testosterone-dependent regulatory hierarchy of the secondary sex-determining mechanism. If there is a master regulatory gene product analogous in its role to testis-organizing H-Y antigen of the primary sex-determining mechanism, one can fairly well predict details of the syndrome caused by its mutational deficiency. for obvious reasons, such a mutation is not expected to affect overtly the sexual development of homozygous females. Affected males should also show no defect in the initial testicular organogenesis, for this process is under the direction of the H-Y antigen. Accordingly, the antimüllerian hormone secreted by testicular Sertoli cells should destroy müllerian ducts. Whether or not any of the gene loci for key sex steroid synthesizing enzymes are included in the testosterone-dependent regulatory hierarchy determines the testosterone synthetic capability of Leydig cells in testes of affected males. At any rate, testosterone synthesis by Leydig cells is an irrelevant side issue, for wolffian ducts, the urogenital sinus, and external genitalia, having been mutationally deprived of their responsiveness to testostosterone, will fail totally in their attempts at masculine differentiation, no matter how high the fetal circulating testosterone level. Consequently, one sees at birth an XY indivudual with undescended testes with the external appearance of a girl but internally lacking extragonadal reproductive organs and ducts of either sex: thus the vagina ends in a blind sac. While a pubertal rise in the circulating testosterone level should have no virilizing effect whatsoever, a greater amount of circulating testosterone means a greater production of estradiol-17β by the microsomal aromatase of extragonadal organs, to which an affected individual is normally responsive. As a result, breasts grow, and an affected adult manifests an overall attractively feminine external appearance.

Apparently have physicians recognized this syndrome in man since the nineteenth century. As many as one in every five human male pseudohermaphrodites encountered in the clinics is said to manifest this specific syndrome (POLANI, 1970), which was defined as the testicular feminization syndrome by MORRIS (1953). Since this defect is invariably transmitted by a heterozygous mother to half of her XY progeny, its X-linked inheritance has long been suspected. The actual proof, however, was obtained in 1975 when two clones of cells (one androgen nonresponsive, and the other normally responsive) were identified on obligatory heterozygotes who are mothers of the affected (MEYER et al., 1975). One or another form of pituitary deficit as well as testicular insufficiencies has, in the past, been suggested as its cause. PRADER (1957) appears to be one of the first to demonstrate the nonresponsiveness to androgen as the cause of Tfm. Probably because axillary as well as pubic hair growth is an androgen-dependent process in both sexes of man, patients with the complete form of this syndrome lack hair growth in these areas. PRADER (1957) found that repeated testosterone-ointment treatments of the patient's pubic area failed to elicit the androgen-dependent hair growth. His claim of androgen-nonresponsiveness as the cause has now been amply substantiated. As to the cause of this nonresponsiveness, the excitement created by the discovery of 5α-dihydrotestosterone (BRACHOVSKY and WILSON, 1968a). understandably produced the notion 5α-reductase deficiency was the cause of this syndrome. In view of the "penis at 12" syndrome discussed in the previous chapter, this notion is now of historical interest only. Nevertheless, it is of some importance to point out that 5α-reductase in many mouse androgen target organs is normally inducible by androgens: thus it becomes noninducible in testicular feminized mice.

Inasmuch as the Tfm syndrome has also been identified in cattle and the dog, there were sufficient causes to suspect that this mutation may in fact identify the master regulatory locus that governs the secondary sex-determining meachanism of mammals (INHORN and OPITZ, 1968). What remained to be done was to identify the same mutation in laboratory animals and see if this apparent point mutation of the single locus confers the androgen-nonresponsiveness to every androgen target organ and cell type of the mammalian body. If the above proved to be the case, one could then identify this master regulatory gene product.

a) Tfm/Y Mice and Rats and Their Fetal Secondary Sex Differentiation

The *Tfm* mutation has indeed been recovered in the rat (ALLISON et al., 1965), and the affected animals came to be known as Stanley-Gumbreck hermaphroditic rats. In the mouse, LYON and HAWKES (1970) established a close linkage of their newly discovered Tfm gene to two previously known X-linked coat structure and color genes, Ta (Tabby) and Blo (Blotchy)). Thus, they were the first to confirm the long suspected X-linkage of the mammalian Tfm locus. In view of this confirmation, affected individuals shall henceforth be identified as Tfm/Y, and their heterozygous mother as Tfm/+. Because of its X-linkage, the body of a Tfm/+ heterozygote is a varying micture of androgen-nonresponsive Tfm cells and normally responsive wild-type + cells.

In 1970, C.W. Bardin's group and mine began independent, as well as many cooperative, systematic studies of Tfm/Y rats and mice. In retrospect, the studies on Tfm/Y mice proved more informative than those on Stanley-Gumbreck rats for the following reasons: (1) Adult Tfm/Y mice possessed two more target organs to be studied than Tfm/Y rats: the submaxillary salivary glands and the kidney. (2) In the rat, which has no X-linked marker genes, only the progeny test distinguished Tfm/+ females from +/+ female rats. Furthermore, affected Tfm/Y, in appearance, resembled the preceding two types of females. In the mouse, by contrast, the use of X-linked coat marker genes, Ta and Blo, enabled us to identify all the expected types in the progeny. For example, a mating between a + Ta +/Y male and a Tfm + Blo/+/+ + female produced a wild-type coat + + +/Y male, Blo hemizygous Tfm + Blo/Y phenotypic females, Blo-varieg ated, Ta-striped Tfm + Blo/+ Ta + heterozygous females and Ta striped + + +/+ Ta + females that no longer carried the Tfm gene. (3) Tfm/+ heterozygous mice were convertible to males by an autosomal dominant Sxr gene, repeatedly mentioned in Part II (CATTANACH et al., 1971). These mosaic males in which Tfm clones and + clones coexisted were extremely useful in identifying responsible cell types in various androgen target organs.

In view of the above, I shall confine most of my discussion to the Tfm mutation of the mouse with only occasional references to that of rats. The findings in these two species were essentially identical, as summarized by Bardin (BARDIN et al., 1973). Circulating testosterone levels of adult Tfm/Y mice as well as the rat were found to be subnormal. In our stock of mice, the mean value was 1.3 ng/ml for

Tfm/Y as compared with 5.9 ng/ml for their +/Y brothers (OHNO et al., 1974). The cause was found in the subnormal activity of 17β-hydroxy steroid dehydrogenase in Tfm/Y testes in the rats (SCHNEIDER and BARDIN, 1970).

If we discount the known deleterious effect of the undescended state on testicular steroid synthesis, the above simply means that testicular Leydig cells of rodents represent one type of androgen target cell and that the above-noted enzyme is normally inducible by testosterone, and that, consequently, it became noninducible in Tfm/Y. However, I should point out that the 1:3 ng/ml testosterone level found in our adult Tfm/Y mice is not really subnormal in the absolute sense, for normal adult males of certain inbred strains such as C57Bl/10, make do with a comparable testosterone level. Our stock of mice, in which the Tfm mutation is maintained, has been selected for extremely aggressive behavior by adult males. The high testosterone level of 5.9 ng/ml seen in our +/Y males might be a reflection of this selection. In contrast, C57Bl/10 males are very peaceful creatures.

The first obvious experiment to do with Tfm/Y mutants was to expose them continuously throughout their early fetal development to high concentrations of exogenous 5α-dihydrotestosterone, because the complete lack of masculine differentiation of their wolffian ducts as well as of the urogenital sinus and external genitalia under this artifical condition would prove once and for all that the testicular feminized phenotype is caused by a mutationally acquired nonresponsiveness of the pertinent fetal target organs to androgens. Apparent deficiencies of their 5α-reductase and testosterone synthesizing capacity fade into the background as mere consequences of a mutation-caused target cell nonresponsiveness. When pregnant Tfm/+ mothers were administered daily with 2 mg of 5α-dihydrotestosterone starting on the 12th postgestational day, their +/+ daughters demonstrated the coexistence of a complete set of male and female extragonadal reproductive organs. This caused considerable postpubertal discomfort to masculinized +/+ females. As their masculine external genitalia blocked the discharge, their uterus began to bloat with progressively accumulating fluid. Yet, the phenotype of their Tfm/Y sibs was not affected in the slightest. The same finding has been reported by GOLDSTEIN and WILSON (1972).

In the previous chapter, it was noted that severance of the connection between the nipple and underlying mammary glands constitutes one of the androgen-induced fetal masculine developents in the mouse. Needless, to say, Tfm/Y mice are invariably endowed with the feminine type of conspicuous nipples. Combining the technique of heteroplastic recombination, noted in the previous chapter, with that of organ cultures in the presence of androgens, KRATOCHWIL and SCHWARTZ (1976) proved that mesenchymal cells are entirely responsible for this fetal androgen action; the combination between Tfm/Y epidermal cells of the nipple-forming area and +/Y or +/+ mesenchymal cells of the corresponding area responded to androgens and yielded the inconspicuous masculine nipple. In contrast, the converse combination proved totally androgen resistant, and it proceeded to develop the conspicuous feminine nipple and underlying mammary glands.

The notion that fetal masculine differentiation is determined by mesenchymal androgen responsiveness, entertained in the previous chapter and illustrated schematically in Fig. 25, found further support in the following observation made on sex-reversed Tfm/+, Sxr- mosaic males. One of the more striking findings was that androgen-nonresponsive Tfm cells of wolffian ducts, which should have perished during early fetal development, were found in goodly numbers among epiidymal epithelial cells of these mosaic males (DREWS et al., 1974). This was obviously due to the so-called metabolic cooperation with neighboring androgen-responsive + cells. The fact that as many as 500 Tfm-epithelial cells may constitute a local clone effectively ruled out the possibility of metabolic help coming from adjacent + epithelial cells for the simple reason of distance. There had to be a sufficient number of + fibroblasts in the underlying mesenchyme that were sustaining their survival. Subsequently, DREWS and DREWS (1975) showed that in response to administered androgens, these Tfm-epithelial cells of epididymis divided as often as adjacent + epithelial cells and that this was the sole reason for their persistence to early adulthood despite continuous death among them. Fig. 28 illustrates this point. There remains little doubt that the mitotic stimulation of epithelial cells of the wolffian duct and probably also of the urogenital sinus so essential to their fetal masculine differentiation, are supplied by androgen-responsive mesenchymal cells. By depriving mesenchymal cells of their androgen responsiveness, the Tfm mutation, in fact, manages to suppress the entire process of fetal masculine differentiation in the presence of H-Y antigen-organized testes.

b) Tfm Mutation and the Neonatal Masculinization of the Central Nervous System

Chapter II discussed different evidences that support the view that neonatal masculine imprinting of the central nervous system of the male rodent is not carried out by either testosterone or by 5α-dihydrotestosterone but by estradiol-17β con-

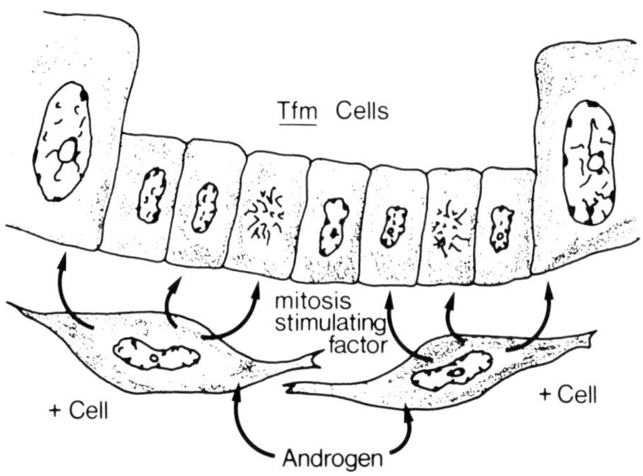

Fig. 28. A schematic illustration of metabolic cooperation between androgen nonresponsive Tfm epithelial cells and underlying wild-type + mesenchymal cells that enabled large patches of Tfm epithelial cells to survive in the epididymis of sex-reversed Tfm/+,Sxr/− males (DREWS and DREWS, 1975). Each patch, often consisting of a few hundred cells, was too large to be helped by adjacent [+]epithelial cells. Androgen-induced mitotic activities were the sole reason for their survival. Mitotic stimuli of androgen-nonresponsive Tfm epithelial cells had to come from underlying wild-type mesenchymal cells, which produced a epithelial cell mitotic stimulating factor in response to androgens

verted *in situ* from testosterone by microsomal aromatase. The enzymatic conversion process from androstenedione to estrone as well as from testosterone to estradiol-17β is illustrated schematically in Fig. 29. Inasmuch as 5α-dihydrotestosterone cannot be aromatized by this enzyme, one should expect that this otherwise most potent androgen is incapable of neonatally masculinizing the central nervous system. This was indeed found to be so (McDONALD and DOUGHTY, 1974). Although opinions on this subject are by no means unanimous, our own experience agrees very well with that reported by McDonald and Doughty.

It appears probable that this particular aspect of the secondary sex-determining mechanism remains unaffected by the Tfm mutation, so that adult Tfm/Y mice are endowed with the masculine imprinted central nervous system. At this point, however, one should recall the very subnormal circulating testosterone levels of adult Tfm/Y. Their neonatal levels might also be subnormal, although mouse

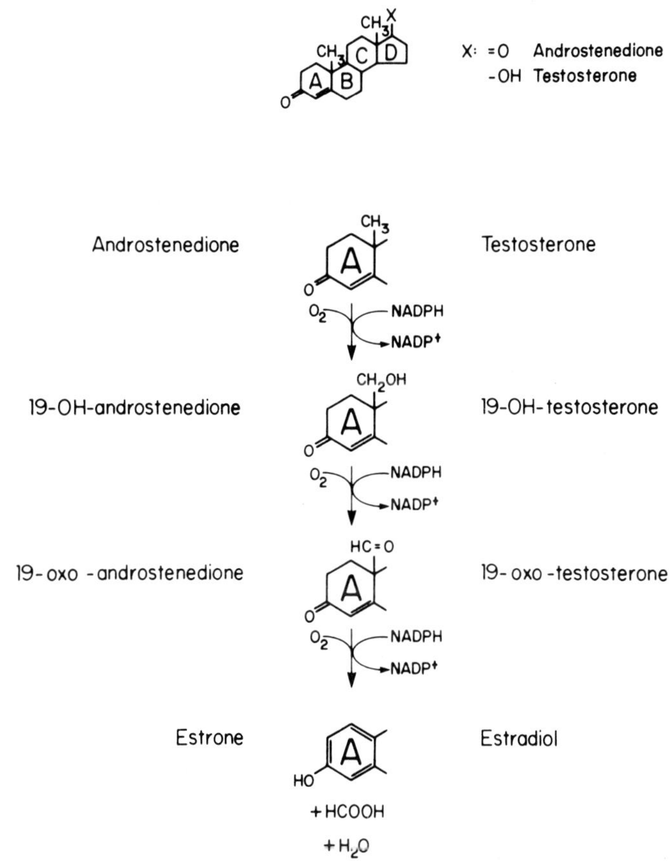

Fig. 29. Schematic illustration of the three-step conversion from androstenedione to estrone (*left*) as well as from testosterone to estradiol-17β (*right*) by the microsomal cytochrome P-450-requiring aromatase. In the end, a methyl group, representing the 19th carbon and two hydrogens on 1β and 2β positions are removed in the form of formic acid and water to complete aromatization of the ring A. This enzyme is ultimately responsible for the production of estrogens by both sexes. Estrone is converted to estradiol by the same 17β-hydroxylation mechanism that converts androstenedione to testosterone

neonates do not yield enough blood for testosterone measurements. After refining the aromatase assay method (REED and OHNO, 1976), K.C. Reed, in my laboratory, studied aromatase activities of various pertinent regions of the rat brain under different conditions and found this enzyme in certain hypothalamic regions to be normally inducible by androgens. Although the mouse brain was too small for this sort of study, if the same holds true, the neonatal hypothalamus of Tfm/Y mice may not possess enough aromatase for meaningful conversion from testosterone to estradiol.

In view of the pessimistic outlook noted above, it was somewhat of a surprise to find that when J.D. Kan of this laboratory transplanted H-2 compatible ovarian fragments under the kidney capsule of castrated Tfm/Y mice, nearly all of them exhibited the constant estrus syndrome with regard to their vaginal smears as well as ovarian histology (OHNO, 1977a). As far as the abolishment of the estradiol-triggered positive feedback LH release response is concerned, the combination of a possibly subnormal endogenous testosterone level and a low noninduced hypothalamic aromatase level is still sufficient for the task of neonatally imprinting the Tfm/Y hypothalamus. The adult sexual behavior of Tfm/Y mice will be duscussed later.

c) Androgen Target Organs of Adult Tfm/Y

Fig. 30 illustrates the effect of a single 10-mg dose of 5*a*-dihydrotestosterone on kidney proximal tubule cells of castrated males. Female cells respond equally well. Aside from hypertrophy, which causes as much as a 45% increase in the wet kidney weight, spectacular rises in the levels of alcohol dehydrogenase (E.C.1.1.1.1.) residing in the supernatant fraction, and β-glucuronidase (E.C.3.2.1.31) residing in lysosomes, should be noted. The fact that this androgen induction is not indiscriminate is indicated by unaffected levels of another lysosmal enzyme, β-glucosidase. Induced β-glucuronidase is continuously excreted into urine (FISHMAN, 1951), which supports the notion expressed in Chapter II that the kidney of the mouse became an androgen target organ for the sake of masculine pheromone production, although two marker enzymes that we have used may not be the key enzymes in pheromone production. I have also noted that, because of the paucity of 5*a*-reductase, the full induction of the mouse kidney requires the help of exogenously administered androgen, the adult male kidney remaining at about a 30% induced state. With regard to these two marker enzymes, as well as the wet kidney weight, Tfm/Y kidneys were totally noninducible (OHNO and LYON, 1970; DOFUKU et al., 1971a). Thus, the mouse kidney became the first target organ in which mutational nonresponsiveness to androgen was demonstrated in terms of normally inducible structural gene products (Fig. 30).

Submaxillary salivary glands constitute another symbolic androgen target organ of the mouse. Here too the total nonresponsiveness to androgens was shown for organ growth and NGF (nerve growth factor) inducibility (LYON et al., 1973) and, later, protease „D" inducibility in addition (SCHENKEIN et al., 1974).

The adult hypothalamo-pituitary axis can also be considered as one of the androgen target organs. Indeed, Tfm/Y pituitary gonadotrophs hypertrophied in response to administered testosterone, while those of normal males and females

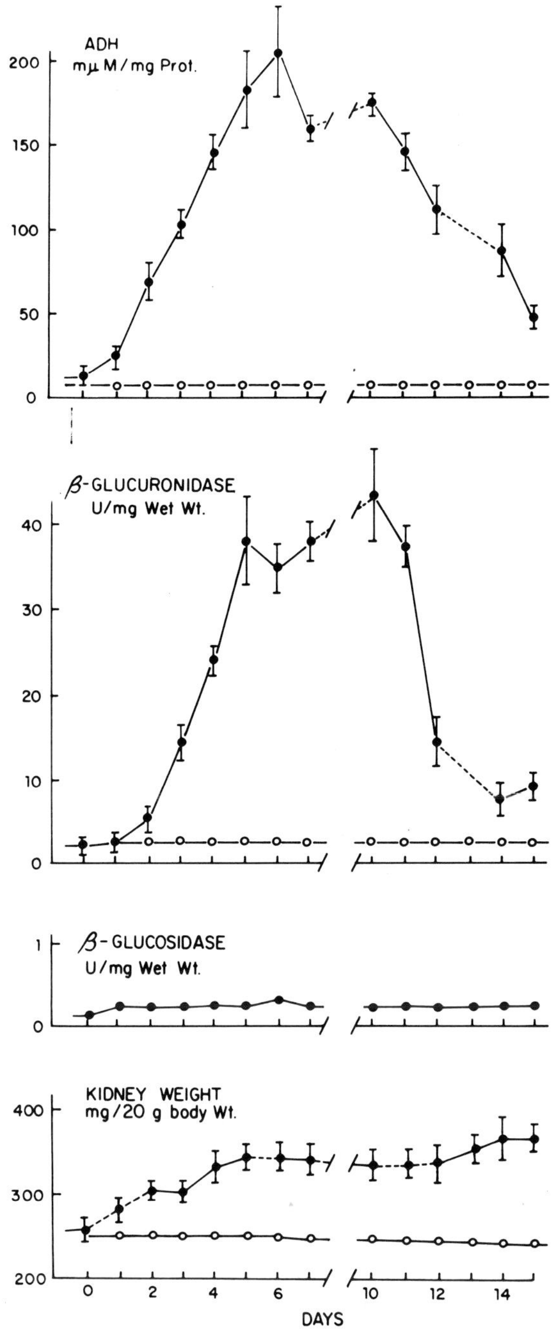

Fig. 30. Induction of ADH (alcohol dehydrogenase), β-glucuronidase, and hypertrophy in the kidney of castrated +/Y male mice (-●-●-) following a single intraperitoneal injection of 10 mg of 5α-dihydrotestosterone contrasted with the total nonresponsiveness shown by Tfm/Y (-○-○-) mice similarly treated (DOFUKU, et al., 1971a). β-glucosidase is used as an example of the structural gene products not affected by androgens

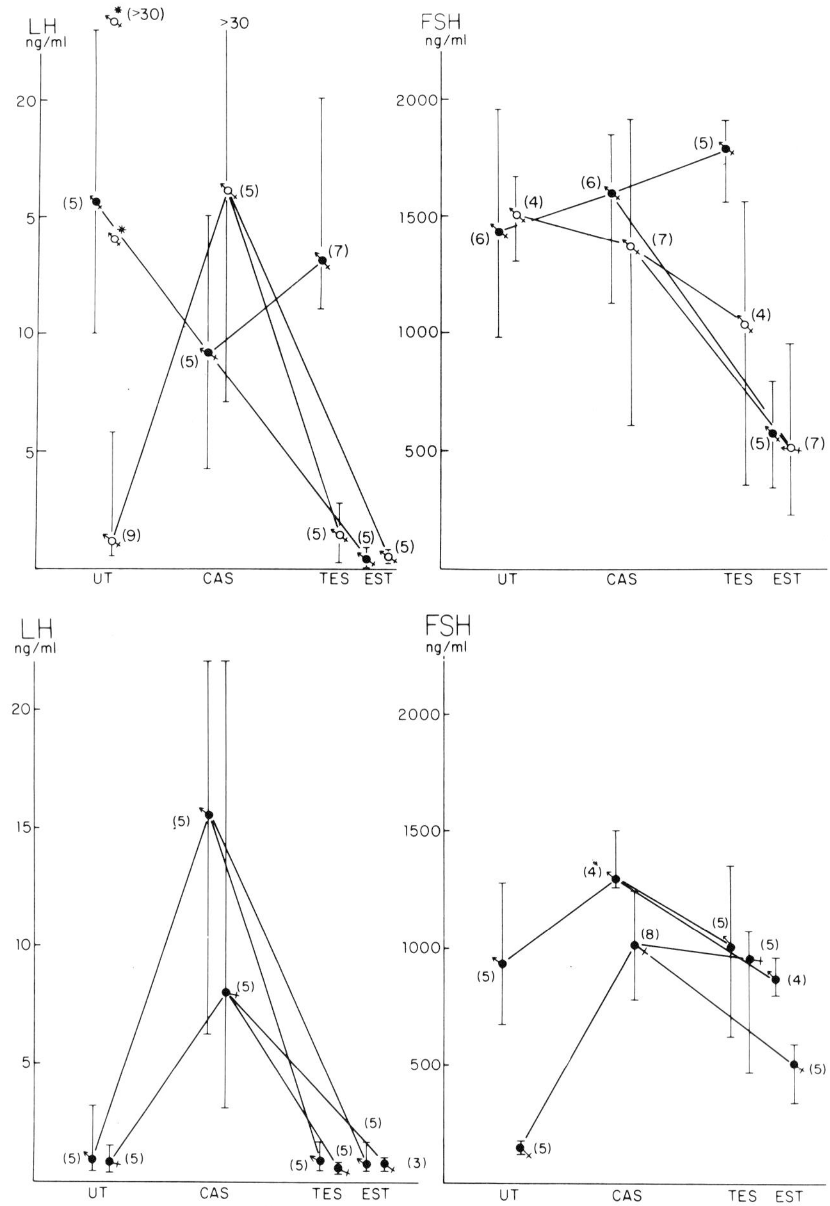

Fig. 31. Circulating LH (*left*) *and FSH* (*right*) levels of +/Y males (♂) and +/+ females (♀) rise following castration (*CAS*) because of the removal of negative feedback inhibition by endogenous sex steroids, and fall back to the original untreated (*UT*) levels following the continuous administration of testosterone (*TES*) or estradiol-17β (*EST*), due to the negative feedback inhibition of each upon their hypothalamopituitary axis. This situation (*bottom*)is contrasted with the situation found in Tfm/Y mice (*top*). In ordinary Tfm/Y (⚥) mice, the Tfm mutation specifically abolishes from the affected hypothalamo-pituitary axis, the negative feedback response to circulating androgens, while leaving the estradiol response intact. Thus untreated, their LH as well as FSH levels are very high and castration or continuous administration of testosterone has little or no effect upon these high levels. Estradiol treatments, in contrast, effectively bring down both levels. A curious fact is that the (0hv) mutation of

atrophied (ITAKURA and OHNO, 1973). Circulating levels of sex steroids are controlled by the negative feedback inhibition of gonadotropin release that sex steroids themselves exert upon the hypothalamo-pituitary axis. Thus, in +/Y male as well as +/+ female mice, castration elevates their circulating LH as well as FSH (follicle-stimulating hormone) levels, which can readily be suppressed by subsequent administration of testosterone propionate as well as of estradiol benzoate (5 doses of 1.0 mg each, 3 days apart), as shown in Fig. 31, bottom. In sharp contrast, castration or testosterone propionate administration had little or no effect upon characteristically high LH and FSH levels of Tfm/Y mice, whereas estradiol bensoate was very effective in suppressing abnormally high LH and FSH levels of Tfm/Y mice (Fig. 31, top). Thus, as far as the negative feedback inhibition mechanism was concerned, the mouse hypothalamo-pituitary axis clearly distinguished testosterone from estradiol. Hence, the Tfm mutation selectively abolished testosterone response while leaving the estradiol one intact. I noted earlier that the neonatal masculine imprinting process, which abolishes the positive feedback LH release response of the hypothalamo-pituitary axis to a rising blood estradiol level so essential to the ovulation of adult females, was not abolished by the Tfm mutation. The contrast, made evident between the neonatal and adult hypothalamo-pituitary axis with regard to its androgen sensitivity, further strengthens the notion that the neonatal imprinting process is not really the androgen response but the estradiol response disguised as the former by the target neuron microsomal aromatase.

One unresolved puzzle is the effect that the (0^{hv}) mutation of the nearby controlling element locus exerts upon the expression of the Tfm gene. This (0^{hv}) mutation causes the preferential activation of the (0^{hv}) -carrying X in $(0+)/(0^{hv})$ heterozygotes.
Thus, a considerable portion of Tfm + (O^{HV}) Blo/+ + (0+) +, Sxr/- males, for example, develop to resemble Tfm + Blo/Y hemizygotes in their coat color as well as in their total androgen nonresponsiveness (OHNO et al., 1974a). Its effect on Tfm (0^{hv})/Y is the puzzling one. In contrast to ordinary Tfm/Y, their wolffian duct persists to adulthood in the form of atrophic epididymis and ductus deferens. Yet these organs, as well as their kidney and submaxillary salivary glands, remain totally nonresponsive to administered androgens. Nevertheless, the negative feedback response to testosterone was clearly restored in their hypothalamo-pituitary axis (Fig. 31, top) KAN et al., 1975).

The Tfm mutation also abolishes the negative feedback in hibition by testosterone of pituitary prolactin release. In the mouse, it has been shown that if pups are

---

Fig. 31. (cont.): the nearby controlling locus restores to the *Tfm* (0^{hv})/Y hypothalamo-pituitary axis the negative feedback response to testosterone. Thus, LH and FSH levels of Tfm (0^{hv})/Y (⚥) are affected by castration and by continuous administeration of testosterone as well as of estradiol exactly in the same manner as are those of +/Y and +/+ mice. *UT*: untreated; *CAS*: two weeks after the castration; *TES*: after 5 treatments 3 days apart with 1 mg of testosterone propionate each; *EST*: the same treatments with estradiol benzoate. The number in each *parenthesis* indicates the number of animals used for a measurement. Sheep LH was used as the standard in the heterologous immunoassay for LH, whereas the phylogenetically closer rat FSH was used as the standard for FSH: hence, the great discrepancies in ng/ml values between LH and FSH that are not at all real (KAN et al., 1975) withheld from a nursing mother overnight and then allowed to suckle the next morning, the suckling stimuli signaled the hypothalamo-pituitary axis of the mother to release a massive amount of prolactin (SINHA et al., 1974). Using the homologous immunoassay, J.D. Kan of this laboratory, and Y.N. Sinha, of the laboratory of Vanderlaan, found that daily administration of 1 mg of testosterone propionate each, starting on the day of delivery, completely suppressed this suckling-triggered pituitary prolactin release in nursing mothers. The well-known inhibitory effect of testosterone upon lactation by nursing mothers (TURKINGTON et al., 1968) can now be explained by its action upon the hypothalamo-pituitary axis. When Tfm/+ heterozygous mothers were examined for this aspect of androgen sensitivity, it was found that 5 out of the 23 testosterone-treated heterozygous mothers (21.7%) were impervious to testosterone treatments and continued to exhibit a suckling-triggered massive prolactin release (Table 6) (OHNO 1977c). In this manner, yet another androgen response of the hypothalamo-pituitary axis has been shown to be abolished by the Tfm mutation.

d) Spermatogenesis and Spermiogenesis by Tfm/Y Germ Cells

When it became clear that the Tfm mutation extinguishes every conceivable androgen response by all the target cell types and organs of the mouse body, this mutation became a tool with which the validity of any questionable androgen response could be scrutinized. We have already seen the example of the neonatal masculine imprinting process of the mouse central nervous system. At least a part of the process that causes the constant estrus syndrome is revealed as the estradiol-dependent process disguised as the androgen-dependent one. The same apparently holds true for Tfm/Y rats (SHAPIRO et al., 1975).

In Chap. 9, I described our own experience, whereby the hypogonadism of hpg/hpg male mice, caused by a congenital deficiency of hypothalamic gonadotropic releasing hormone (CATTANACH et al., 1977), was remedied by continuous administration of either testosterone or 5a-dihydrotestosterone. It has long been known that a similar treatment manages to maintain spermatogenesis and

Table 6. *Tfm* mutation abolition of the negative feedback inhibition by testosterone of the suckling-induced pituitary prolactin release by lactating mothers

Tfm/+ ♀	Serum prolactin (ng/ml)		
	No. ♀	Before	After
Untreated	19	31.0	331.4
TES-treated: Responsive	18	8.0	6.9
TES-treated: Resistant	5	83.1	438.4

These *Tfm*/+ heterozygous females were treated daily with 1 mg testosterone propionate for 13 days starting on the day of delivery. Initial blood samples were collected on the morning of the 13th day, after the litter had been removed overnight. The second samples were collected after temporarily starved pups were allowed to suckle for 1 h. The homogolous immune assay was used using mouse prolactin as the standard. A pertinent hypothalamic region or regions of the 5 resistant *Tfm*/+ heterozygous mothers must have effectively been *Tfm*-monoclonal. TES = testosterone. The work of J. D. Kan and N. Y. Sinha (OHNO, 1977c).

spermiogenesis in hypophysectomized male rats. Accordingly, the male germ cell maturation process has customarily been thought of as a definitely androgen-dependent process (STEINBERG 1971). More recently, the finding of a very high affinity androgen-binding protein, which is apparently synthesized and secreted by testicular Sertoli cells into efferent duct fluid (FRENCH and RITZEN, 1973), and of the nuclear-cytosol androgen-receptor protein in seminiferous tubule preparations (HANSSON et al., 1974), was thought to substantiate the androgen dependence of spermatogenesis and spermiogenesis, although exactly how has not been elaborated.

Chapter 9 also introduced the hypothesis of LIFSCHITZ (1972), which postulates the X-inactivation in male germ cells, whereby their sex chromosome constitution becomes OY in the functional sense. Indeed, X elimination during primordial germ cell proliferation conferred the OY constitution upon definitive spermatogonia of one rodent species-Microtus oregoni (OHNO et al., 1963). If X inactivation normally occurs during differentiation of mammalian male germ cells, it is likely to take place in the neonatal testis at the stage where large primordial germ cells transform to much smaller definitive spermatogonia. From this stage onward, male germ cells can live as parasites of Sertoli cells, which protect and nurse them by supplementing genetic deficiencies of male germ cells brought about by the X inactivation. Because of this intimate relationship between postnatal male germ cells and Sertoli cells, the androgen dependence of nursing Sertoli cells can easily be mistaken for that of male germ cells. Furthermore, the Tfm locus being X-linked, one can hardly imagine how male germ cells with the inactivated X can maintain the androgen responsiveness.

When chimeric males were made by the fusion of +/Y with Tfm/Y blastocysts, at least some of them developed as fertile males and transmitted the Tfm gene to some of their progeny (LYON et al., 1975). There remains little doubt that, if nursed by androgen-responsive +/Y Sertoli cells, the Tfm/Y germ line can complete spermatogenesis and spermiogenesis to yield functional spermatozoa. It would appear that the notion of androgen dependence of spermatogenesis and spermiogenesis should be laid to rest for eternity.

e) Asexual Behavior of Adult Tfm/Y

Needless to say, consequences of the neonatal masculine imprinting of the rodent central nervous system extend beyond the mere abolishment from the hypothalamo-pituitary axis of the estradiol-triggered positive feedback LH release response. For example +/+ female mice of our stock, if neonatally imprinted either with testosterone or with estadiol-17β, simultaneously manifest the constant estrus syndrome and masculine behavior upon reaching puberty. No additional introduction of exogenous sex steroids is needed. If properly reared in isolation from normal males as well as from other masculinized females, a masculinized female readily attacks a normal adult male introduced to her cage. In fact, she appears to enjoy the combative advantage over an intruding normal male, for she does not appear to emit aggression-provoking masculine body odor since she is not under the influence of androgen. As far as aggressive masculine behavior is concerned, the only distinguishing characteristic unique to masculinized females is found in their tendency to emit high-pitched squeaks as they engage in combat. Adult +/Y males seldom if ever do this. Masculinized females also mount normal females in estrus. This trait in our mouse stock, however, cannot be considered uniquely masculine, for our normal females in estrus mount each other with considerable frequency.

In contrast, adult Tfm/Y exhibits no trace of masculine behavior, even if the constant estrus syndrome is induced in them by ovarian transplants following castration. Neither do they exhibit feminine behavior.

Human Tfm/Y patients, so attractively feminine in their appearance, are also said to be entirely feminine in their psychological outlook, fulfilling the role of wives and even of mothers toward adopted children without any difficulty (MONEY, 1965; INHORN and OPITZ, 1968). After making certain that the vagina was developed enough to permit a smooth penile intromission, over the years we have kept many a Tfm/Y adult mouse with a normal male overnight. Upon inspection the next morning, we have yet to see a single instance of copulatory plug formation, nor have we ever witnessed a single serious mounting attempt made by an adult male upon a Tfm/Y (OHNO et al., 1974b). The absence of sexual behavior has also been noted in Tfm/Y rats (SHAPIRO et al., 1975). Intact Tfm/Y mice are totally ignored by normal males whereas Tfm/Y in transplanted ovary-induced constant estrus are often viciously attacked by adult males. So far, our attempts to induce either masculine or feminine behavior in Tfm/Y by neonatal and/or postpubertal sex steroid treatments have met with total failure. This puzzling inability of the androgen-nonresponsive Tfm/Y central nervous system to generate any sort of sexual behavior may or may not be of significance in our understanding of the elicitation of sexual behavior.

Because of probably subnormal levels of circulating testosterone as well as hypothalamic microsomal aromatase, pertinent regions in the neonatal Tfm/Y central nervous system may receive an incomplete masculine imprinting. While this is sufficient to cause the postpubertal manifestation of the constant estrus syndrome, other centers pertinent to sexual behavior of the Tfm/Y brain may have become suspended in the half-way imprinted neuter state. If so, the neonatal estradiol treatment of Tfm/Tfm homozygous females should succeed in the complete masculine imprinting of the androgen nonresponsive central nervous system. By mating an already noted chimeric male, producing Tfm spermatozoa, to Tfm/+ heterozygous females, M. F. Lyon has recovered a number of Tfm/Tfm homozygous females that function as normally fertile females, at least in the beginning (LYON et al., 1975).

Chapter 13

The Tfm Mutation Affects the Nuclear-Cytosol Androgen-Receptor Protein

All the pertinent observations made on the androgen responsiveness of Tfm/Y mice and rats were summarized in Chap. 12. As a result, the X-linked Tfm locus emgerged as the master regulatory gene of the secondary (extragonadal) sex-determining meachanism. It can be recalled that in the primary (gonadal) sex-determining meacanism, it was the master regulatory gene product, H-Y antigen, which was unequivocally identified. What remains to be worked out is the genetics of H-Y antigen expression, in which not only the Y but also the X and possibly also an autosome are involved.

In contrast, the story of the secondary sex-determining mechanism is that while the X-linked master regulatory locus has been identified, some doubts remain as to the identity of its product. The Tfm locus in the mammalian genome appears to represent the one and only structural locus for nuclear-cytosol androgen receptor-protein. However, irrevocable proof that a small amount of this receptor protein found in Tfm/Y mice and rats is a mutationally altered protein still remains to be obtained.

When systematic experimental analysis of the Tfm mutation in mice and rats began in 1970, relevant studies on so-called nuclear-cytosol receptor proteins for steroid hormones were also coming into vogue. It soon became apparent that the nuclear-cytosol androgen-receptor protein, at least in its conceptually idealized form, has nearly all the attributes of being the master regulatory gene product of the secondary sex-determining meachanism. Naturally, the possible connection between the two was explored.

The current dogma with regard to how the nuclear-cytosol steroid-receptor protein serves as an instrument of a given steroid hormone in its target cell can be summerized as follows: Probably because of its lipophilic nature, a steroid hormone appears to encounter no serious hindrance in penetrating through the target cell plasma membrane. For this reason, its receptor molecules are found not on the plasma membrane but in the cytosol (supernatant) fraction of the cytoplasm. These receptor proteins, usually existing in the dimeric or even tetrameric form, demonstrate a fittingly high binding affinity to a specific steroid hormone: a dissociation constant (Kd) of 10^{-10} M or thereabout at 0°C. Once bound to its steroid hormone, the new acceptor binding site is created on the receptor molicule *via* an allosteric effect. The steroid-receptor complexes then move into the target cell nucleus, and these molecules seek and bind to a finite number of the acceptor sites present in the genetic apparatus of its target cell. In one way or another, such associations result in the induction of a specific set of structural gene products. We shall now examine various aspects of the above dogma, concentrating our attention upon the nuclear-cytosol androgen-receptor protein only.

a) General Properties of the Nuclear-Cytosol Androgen-Receptor Protein

As noted earlier, the mean serum testosterone level of adult +/Y males of our mouse strain is 5.9 ng/ml, whereas that of adult +/+ females is 0.4 ng/ml (OHNO et al., 1974). This one order of magnitude sexual difference in adult circulating testosterone levels appears to characterize most mammalian species, including our own. Among laboratory mice, however, this difference presents the maximal difference to be found only in high androgen strains such as BALB/C. In low androgen strains such as C57B10, a sexual difference may be as little as four fivefold. Fetal serum testosterone concentrations under which the wolffian duct, urogenital sinus, and external genitalia of the male but not the female have to undergo masculine growth and differentiation, can best be studied in mammals with a long gestation period such as man. During the critical period–roughly between 84 and 140 gestational days–the male androgen level temporarily rises to again create one order of magnitude sexual difference, i.e., a mean of 3.0 ng/ml for the male as opposed to 0.4 ng/ml for the female (REYES et al., 1974). Adult sera of many mammalian species including man contain a class of globulin having a relatively high binding affinity to sex steroids. Its characteristic absence in the mouse might be the main reason that males of low androgen strains do not suffer from androgen insufficiencies as far as their reproductive capacities are concerned. The binding affinity of mouse serum albumin to testosterone is a great deal less than that shown by the above-noted class of globulin of other species.

Nevertheless, the presence or absence of a high-affinity serum testosterone-binding protein is totally irrelevant to the problem created by only one order of magnitude sexual difference in the circulating testosterone level; if anything, its presence tends to reduce more effectively a free testosterone level of the male, thus further diminishing the already meager sex difference.

Inasmuch as we find no sexual difference in the androgen responsiveness of corresponding target cell types, we realize that each target cell type cannot be made too responsive to androgens, for they should remain in the noninduced state at the female level of circulating testosterone. Furthermore, even at the adult male testosterone level, only those organs that are essential for male reproduction can afford to acquire the fully induced state, e. g., the wolffian duct and urogenital sinus derivatives. In sharp contrast, their raison d'etre dictates that symbolic androgen target organs of sexually dimorphic species should remain only in a partially induced state, as the mouse kidney indeed does, at the base testosterone level charateristic of adult males. Only then can they show further response to the greater than normal increases in the testosterone level triggered by the elation of combative victories over rival males as well as by the anticipation of sexual intercourse. Indeed, when a bull is teased by being led up to a cow, an immediate release of pituitary LH occurs. As a result, his testosterone level rises from 4 ng/ml to 19 ng/ml in 1.5 h (KATONGOLE et al., 1971). Apparently due to a similar mechanism, the rate of beard growth of a man increases in anticipation of meeting a girl friend following a period of abstinence (ANON, 1970).

I believe that the above are the very reasons for the apparent absence of the membrane-bound receptor in all the androgen target cell types, as well as for the limited occurrence of 5α-reductase among the androgen target organs, for both of them tend to make androgen target cell types overly sensitive to circulating testosterone. I have previously remarked that, in a number of androgen target organs of the mouse, 5α-reductase became one of the enzymes to be induced by androgens. Now, we can appreciate the cleverness of this evolutionary strategy. By placing the 5α-reductase locus under the control of the Tfm locus, those androgen target cell types are made to remain relatively insensitive at low circulating testosterone concentrations while becoming supersensitive in the normal male environment. Conversely, by giving a high constitutive level to 5α-reductase, an androgen target cell type can be made responsive to a low adult female level of testosterone. Indeed, hairlessness of a complete form of Tfm/Y women reveals the axillary as well as pubic hair growth of adult women to be an androgen-dependent process.

The cytosol androgen-receptor protein of the mouse and other mammalian species is detected as a tritiated androgen-bound 8.5S peak in the sedimentation profile after glycerol or sucrose gradient centrifugation. At a high salt concentration of 0.5 M KC 1, these 8.5S polymers dissociate and reappear as a 4.5S subunit peak (Fig. 32, left). Each subunit apparently has at least one androgen-binding site, and there is an indication that suggests that this subunit molecule has a rod-like shape. During the incubation process, a tritiated androgen used as a probe may be metabolized by enzymes depicted in Fig. 27 that contaminate the cytosol fraction. Since divergent patterns of androgen metabolism characterize individual target organs, if one is not aware of possible enzymatic conversions of a probe,

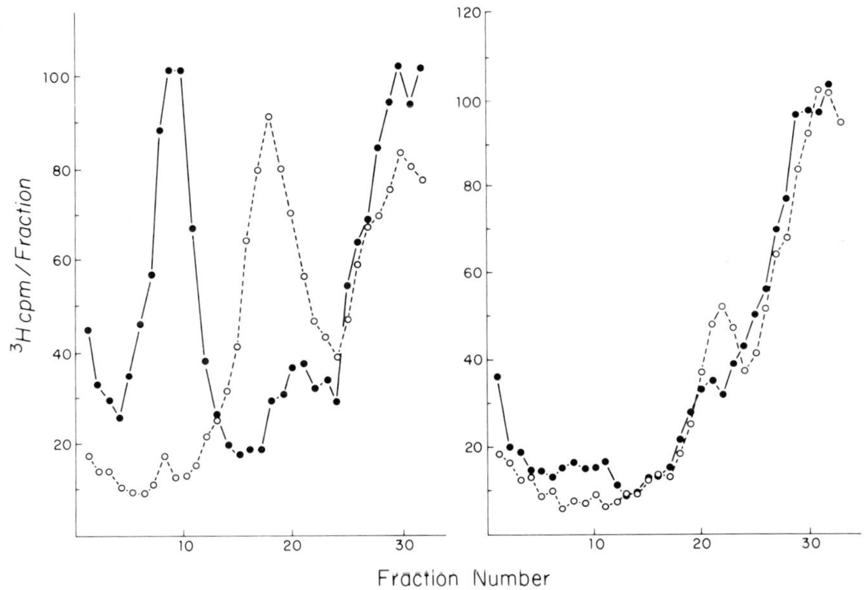

Fig. 32. Linear glycerol gradient (5% – 35%) analysis of the brain cytosol incubated with 5 x 10^{-9} *M* tritiated 5α-dihydrotestosterone. +/+ female (*left*) is compared with Tfm/Y (*right*). Centrifugation took place in a SW 50.1 rotor at 216,000 *g* for 15 h at 2 °C. Direction of sedimentation is from *right* to *left*. The 8 – 9 S peak of the nuclear-cytosol androgen receptor, in its presumably native state, is centered around fractions 9 – 10 (-●-●-). In high salt (0.5 M KC1), androgen receptors dissociated into subunits forming the 4 – 5S peak (-○-○-). A residual presence of androgen receptor in Tfm/Y is more readily discernible as a dissociated subunit peak. Each fraction underwent charcoal treatment before counting (ATTARDI et al., 1976)

one can easily be misled to believe in the existence of a few different kinds of organ-specific androgen-receptor proteins. Not surprisingly, in addition to the 5α-dihydrotestosterone-receptor protein found in the rat prostate (BRUCHOVSKY and WILSON, 1968b; MAINWARING, 1969; BAULIEU and JUNG, 1970), the testosterone receptor had been reported in rat levator ani muscle (JUNG and BAULIEU, 1972) as well as in the mouse kidney (BARDIN et al., 1973), and discrete anabolic and androgenic steroid receptors in rat skeletal muscle (STEINITZ et al., 1971).

In sharp contrast, our own experience with the mouse from the very beginning (GEHRING et al., 1971) has been always to find the same androgen-receptor protein in all the divergent target organs (ATTARDI and OHNO, 1974; ATTARDI et al., 1976; ATTARDI and OHNO, 1976). After knowing the characteristic pattern of androgen metabolism peculiar to each target organ, if care is taken to minimize contamination of the cytosol fraction with androgen-metabolizing enzymes of Fig. 27, for example by centrifuging the homogenate at 216,000*g* for 60 min (ATTARDI and OHNO, 1974), we found that regardless of the origin with regard to organ, age, and sex, the nuclear cytosol androgen receptor-protein of the mouse invariably demonstrated the highest binding affinity to 5α-dihydrotestosterone. In addition, however, it showed 50% as much binding affinity to testosterone and also, quite surprisingly, a binding affinity to estradiol-17β, although one order of magnitude less (ATTARDI et al., 1976). Despite its supereffectiveness as an androgenic inducer on the rat embryonic wolffian duct (SCHULTZ and WILSON, 1974) as well as on the mouse kidney (OHNO, et al., 1971), the mouse nuclear-cytosol androgen-receptor protein showed no binding affinity whatsoever to 5α-androstan-3α, 17β-diol. This is the very reason for believing that its superefficacy is due to its efficient *in situ* reverse conversion to 5α-dihydrotestosterone (see Fig. 27).

As to measurements of the exact binding affinity to each of the relevant steroids noted above, an underestimation is inherent in the method, for separation of the bound from the free form of steroid molecules, either by gradient centrifugation or by charcoal absorption, creates a nonequilibrium state. With regard to the binding affinity to 5α-dihydrotestosterone, a much greater cause of underestimation was found in a conversion by the second enzyme of Fig. 27 of a tritiated probe to 5α-androstandiol, to which the receptor has no affinity. Despite all the precautions, the above inevitably occurr ed in the kidney cytosol even at 0°C. We found the adult brain cytosol to contain the least amount of the undesirable enzyme. For this reason, we believe that the Kd of $0.8 \pm 0.1 \times 10^{-9}$M for 5α-dihydrotestosterone, obtained on the brain cytosol, is the closest approximation of the true binding affinity of the nuclear cytosol androgen receptor-protein to this most potent androgen (ATTARDI et al., 1976); accordingly, $1.0 - 2.0 \times 10^{-9}$ M is the Kd for testosterone and 8.0×10^{-9} M as that for estradiol-17β.

The tacit assumption during earlier stages of steroid-receptor studies was that only *bona fide* target cell types and organs of a particular steroid hormone should be endowed with the specific receptor of that steroid. Earlier works appeared to have substantiated this generally held belief (MAINWARING and MANGAN, 1973). The ubiquitous expression of steroid hormone receptors in general, and sex steroid receptors in particular, however, soon became apparent. Thus, the nuclear-cytosol androgen-receptor was identified in human fibroblasts obtained from skin biopsies from presumably androgen-sensitive as well as nonsensitive regions of men and women (KEENAN et al., 1974). Similarly, androgen as well as estrogen receptors were found in an established mouse fibroblast line (JUNG-TESTAS et al., 1976). While the hypothalamus-preoptic area of the brain can be considered as the legitimate androgen target region, it takes a great deal of imagination to accept the androgen dependence of the cerebral cortex. Yet, in the mouse brain of both sexes, the cerebral cortex as a whole contained 20% - 80% as many androgen receptors as the hypothalamic preoptic area (ATTARDI and OHNO, 1976). Previously reported anabolic steroid-specific receptors found in rat skeletal muscle (STEINITZ et al., 1971) have since been identified as the ordinary nuclear-cytosol androgen-receptor protein with the general properties just defined (MICHEL and BAULIEU, 1974).

The mouse kidney, while an authentic androgen target, can hardly be thought of as an estrogen target, for a massive dose of estradiol brings about a barely perceptible response. Yet, estradiol receptors were as prominent as androgen receptors in the mouse kidney of both sexes (BULLOCK and BARDIN, 1975). In fact, I cannot think of a single mouse organ that is totally devoid of the nuclear-cytosol androgen-receptor protein.

This ubiquitous expression of the nuclear cytosol androgen receptor-protein immediately reminds us of the equally ubiquitous expression of testis-organizing H-Y antigen – the master regulatory gene product of the primary sex-determining mechanism. As discussed in Part II, such ubiquitous expression is rather expected of the master regulatory gene product. While the expression of H-Y antigen was fittingly male specific, no sexual difference whatsoever has been observed in the expression of nuclear cytosol androgen receptor in all the cell types and organs examined (Fig. 33). This attests to the oft repeated fact that the secondary sex-determining mechanism of mammals is not at all based on a sexual difference in the genetic constitution.

Faced with the rather ubiquitous expression of androgen receptors, one might be tempted to attribute a difference between the target and nontarget cell types to a great difference in numbers of androgen receptors per cell. The extreme dubiousness of this notion shall soon become apparent. While it is true that adult male accessory reproductive organs (seminal vesicles, prostates, etc.) contain vast numbers of androgen receptrors, it should be realized that castration causes these organs to undergo progressive atrophy until they become truly microscopic in size. Accordingly, androgens act upon these organs not only to cause the specific induction of enzymes and proteins, which is the epithelial response, but also to cause rapid organ growth by mitotic activities of epithelial cells, which has been defined as the mesenchymal response (see Fig. 25 and 28). Thus, in these organs, one is encountering the combination of two responses that are independent of each other. From the observation schematically illustrated in Fig. 28, it has been established that the presence of the nuclear-cytosol androgen-receptors within epithelial cells is not required for their androgen-induced mitotic activities, for the mitosis-stimulating factor emanates from underlying mesenchymal cells in response to androgens (DREWS and DREWS, 1975). For which of the two responses is so great a number of androgen receptors required, even if such a requirement exists? A substantial proportion of the cells constituting a rapidly growing population is in the S and G2 phases. If the androgen-receptor gene has a pe-

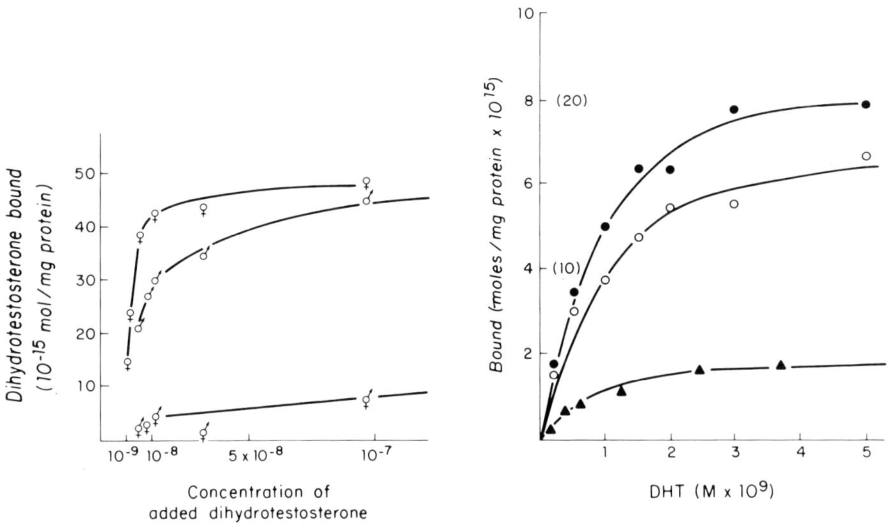

Fig. 33. Specific androgen binding as a function of added 5α-dihydrotestosterone is compared between castrated +/Y males (♂ or ○), +/+ females (♀ or ●), and Tfm/Y (⚥ or ▲) in the kidney cytosol (*left*) and the brain cytosol (*right*). In both organs, +/+ females demonstrated a higher androgen receptor level than castrated +/Y males. Although males were castrated 9 days earlier, a still persisting residual androgen might have interfered. Exactly the same degree of androgen-receptor deficiency is seen in both organs of TFM/Y, although the two sets of data are derived from our publications 5 years apart (GEHRING et al., 1971; ATTARDI et al., 1976). In order to calculate a low affinity but high capacity steroid binding at each concentration has to be subtracted from each value of the above

culiar propensity to be transcribed more efficiently during these two phases, vast numbers of androgen receptors contained in these organs may merely reflect the consequence of androgen-induced cell proliferation. Indeed, it has been known that the number of androgen receptors in these organs rapidly declines following castration (BAULIEU and JUNG, 1970; MAINWARING and MANGAN, 1973).

In contrast, androgens elicit from the mouse kidney a purely epithelial response, for no mitotic proliferation is included in the response. Yet, proximal tubule cells are markedly affected by androgen, and a pronounced hypertrophy of individual epithelial cells is accompanied by nearly 100-fold induction of specific marker enzymes (see Fig. 26 and 30). How many androgen receptors per cell are required for so remarkable an androgen response? Even if we make the assumption that only proximal tubule cells, the real androgen target cell type, of the kidney are endowed with the nuclear-cytosol androgen-receptor protein, the number that we come up with is 1500 - 2000 androgen-binding sites (receptor subunit molecules?) per cell (ATTARDI and OHNO, 1974; OHNO, 1976c). In view of the recently discussed ubiquitous expression of sex steroid receptors, such an assumption is probably unwarranted. It follows then that as far as the specific induction of enzymes and proteins – the purely epithelial response – is concerned, the required number of androgen-receptor subunits per cell may be no more than several hundred. So small a number is satisfying, if one realizes that each *Escherichia coli* is endowed with no more than 10 molecules of the famous *lac*-repressor protein.

Finally, we have to deal with the ultimate question of exactly how androgen-bound receptors in the target cell nucleus manage to induce the selective synthesis of a specific set of enzymes and proteins? So much work has been done in this particular area of the steroid-receptor field to yield so little information. All the studies of binding between steroid-bound receptors and the genomic DNA as well as the target chromatin fraction were based on the assumption that the hypothetical acceptor site in the target cell nucleus must necessarily represent, either directly or indirectly, the *operator* DNA base sequence of each inducible structural gene. When one deals with the purely epithelial response (parenchymal response in the case of liver), this assumption in its bare essence must be correct. Developmentally more important steroid hormone actions during fetal growth, such as androgen-induced growth and masculine differentiation of the embryonic wolffian duct and urogenital sinus, on the other hand, have been established as the purely mesenchymal response (CUHNA, 1972; KRATCHWILL and SCHWARTZ, 1976). In my experience, mesenchymal cells of androgen target organs, either *in vivo* or *in vitro*, demonstrate no appreciable response to administered androgens. All they do, apparently is to release the hypothetical epithelial cell mitotic-stimulating factor into their immediate vicinity (see Fig. 25 and 28). Whether the nuclear translocation of androgen-bound receptor is relevant for such a release may even be questioned.

Going back to the purely epithelial response, which should be studied on epithelial nuclei only, the notion cherished until a few years ago (that histones are the general utility repressors of gene expression so that their removal from a specific stretch of DNA by one or the other of the so-called nonhistone acidic proteins constitutes the act of gene activation) has been shattered by the ubiquitous presence of nucleosomes. The equally naive notion (equating the cytoplasmic *messenger* RNA with a faithful transcript of its structural gene in its near-entirety) has also been shattered by the recent identification of huge precursors of cytoplasmic *messenger* RNAs among the so-called heterogeneous nuclear RNAs. Since all these points have been discussed in Chap. 4, nor more shall be said of the many claimed proofs of the postulated binding between the acceptor site on the genomic DNA and the acceptor binding site of steroid hormone-bound receptors. At any rate, my personal prejudice has always been to favor post transcriptional control, i. e., stabilization of a ubiquitously expressed huge transcript so that it can be processed to emerge as cytoplasmic *messenger* RNA instead of suffering instant degradation inside the nucleus. Indeed, steroid-bound receptors that seem to bind to nearly all things have also been found in association with nuclear ribonucleo proteins (LIAO et al., 1973).

Uncertainty about the exact mode of action of the nuclear-cytosol androgen-receptor protein, however, should not hinder us from identifying the expected class of mutations that affect the inducibility by androgen of each structural gene in the target epithelial nucleus. Each of these structural genes that are normally inducible by androgen in one or the other of the androgen target organs has to be equipped with the recognition signal (base sequence) by which the androgen-bound receptor protein can single out that particular gene from the multitudes as the one to induce. Whether this is done directly by the receptor or indirectly through another protein is immaterial, and so is the question of whether this sequence is recognized as DNA of a gene or as RNA of the gene's fresh transcript. We shall define this base sequence as the operator of an androgen-inducible structural gene. The point here is that just as the androgen-receptor locus can mutate to specify a mutant receptor that can be either superefficient or functionally defunct, so can the operator of each androgen-inducible structural gene mutate to change its expression in a pertinent target cell type from inducible to either non-inducible or constitutive.

What would be the phenotype expected of the operator noninducible (0^s) mutation of a given androgen-inducible structural gene? Genetically, such a mutation should map either very close to or within the affected structural gene, and since the 0^s mutation can only show *cis* expression, operationally it should be recognized as a recessive. +/Y or +/+ mice that are $0^s/0^s$ homozygous should exhibit all other normal androgen responses. Abnormality should be seen only in the target epithelial cell type in which the wild type of 0^s is normally androgen inducible. The noninducibility should be confined to one protein or enzyme specified by the 0^s gene, while all other normally inducible proteins and enzymes should remain unaffected. Needless to say, Tfm representing a defunct mutation of the master regulatory locus should be totally epistatic over the 0^s mutation of a mere structural gene. As illustrated in Fig. 34, we identified such a mutation of the β-glucuronidase locus in our stock of mice (DOFUKU et al., 1971, a, b).

The noninducible phenotype was associated with an electrophoretic variant of β-glucuronidase (Fig. 34, top), thus establishing either the close linkage or identity between the 0^s mutation and the enzyme structural gene. Its phenotype was operationally recessive. In $0^s/0^s$ homozygous +/Y males as well as +/+ females, the constitutive expression of this enzyme in other organs was not at all affected. In the androgen-induced kidney, too, the degree of induction of ADH as well as hypertrophy was normal. The induced level of β-glucuronidase, however, was barely above the base noninducible level. In $0^s/0^s$ homozygous Tfm/Y, even this barely perceptible induction of a mutant β-glucuronidase was totally abolished (Fig. 34, bottom). In 1973, either an identical or very similar mutation of this enzyme locus was described in other strains of the mouse (SWANK et al., 1973).

An alternative to the above, the operator constitutive mutation has been identified on the Slp lucus of the mouse situated in the middle of the H-2 region. As illustrated in Fig. 17, Ss and Slp are very closely linked. Ss was originally found as a genetically polymorphic serum protein by SHREFFLER and OWEN (1963). It has recently been shown that the Ss locus actually specifies one of the complements, most likely C4 (LACHMAN et al., 1975; CURMAN et al., 1975). Shreffler's view on the nearby Slp locus is that it is a duplicate of the Ss gene that became considerably more androgen dependent than the original by acquiring a more efficient operator site for the nuclear-cytosol androgen-receptor protein. In the C3H.0H strain, for example, the adult male serum levels of Ss and Slp are 0.9 and 0.8 standard units, while the corresponding values for the female are 0.4 and 0. Tfm/Y of C3H.0H background demonstrate no detectable Slp before or after androgen treatment, whereas Slp is androgen inducible in their +/+ sisters (HANSEN and SHREFFLER, 1976). When Ss^{w7} allele isolated from a Slp-positive wild female by J. KLEIN (1975) was introduced into C3H, +/+ females as well as Tfm/Y of this new C3H.W7 strain congenic to C3H.0H demonstrated high constitutive serum Slp levels of 1.86 and 1.71 standard units (HANSEN and SHREFFLER, 1976).

The successful identification of both postulated types of operator mutations affecting two unlinked structural gene loci that are under the control of the X-linked Tfm locus gives us a renewed hope that as far as the epithelial response is concern-

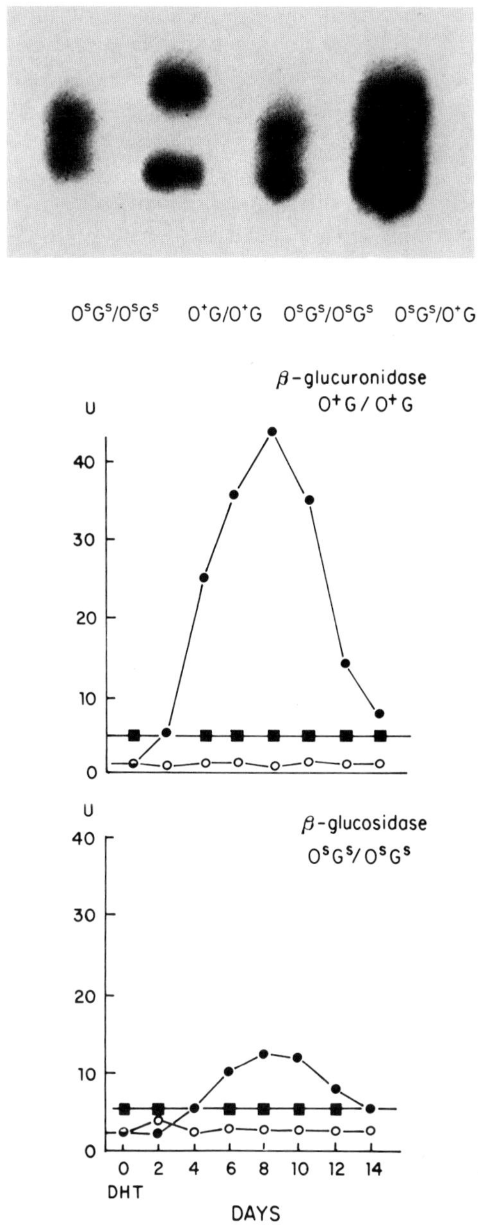

Fig. 34. An *operator noninducible* (0^s) mutation of the mouse β-glucuronidase locus is characterized as to its most pertinent properties.
Top: Electrophoretic phenotypes of β-glucuronidase from liver of $0^s/0^s$ homozygotes (*Slots 1* and *3*), wild-type homozygote (*slot 2*), and heterozygote (*slot 4*). The anodal direction is *upward*.
Bottom: The inducibility of wild-type β-glucuronidase (*top*) ist compared with that of $0^s/0^s$-homozygous enzyme in the kidney of castrated +/Y males following a single 1.0 mg dose of 5α-dihydrotestosterone (-●-●-). The constitutive enzyme level in liver is also shown (-■-■-). In androgen-treated Tfm/Y mice, both enzymes remained noninducible (-○-○-) (DOFUKU et al., 1971a, and b)

ed, the exact mode of action of the nuclear-cytosol androgen-receptor protein shall soon be revealed. If both wild-type and operator mutated structural genes noted above can be cloned in E. coli, the true binding study with androgen-receptor complexes can then be performed.

b) Deficiency of the Nuclear-Cytosol Androgen-Receptor Protein Shown in Affected Tfm/Y

Earlier studies done between 1969 and 1972 have certainly indicated that mammalian tissues might contain several different kinds of androgen receptors: 5α-dihydrotestosterone receptor, testosterone receptor, anabolic androgen receptor, etc. More recent studies noted in the preceding section, on the contrary, have increasingly favored my original notion that there is only one species of the nuclear-cytosol androgen receptor-protein in the mammalian body (OHNO, 1971). While this receptor demonstrates the highest binding affinity to 5α-dihydrotestosterone (Kd = $0.8 + 0.1 \times 10^{-9}$, ist binding affinity to testosterone itself is half as strong. Accordingly, in those target cell types that characteristically lack 5α-reductase, this receptor can function quite well utilizing testosterone itself as an inducer.

Contrary to the original belief in the target cell type-specific occurence, the expression of this nuclear-cytosol androgen-receptor turned out to be not only ubiquitous but also constitutive, the same receptor level being found in the corresponding cell types of males and females (Fig. 33). This finding clearly suggested that the receptor gene locus is not under the control of another regulatory locus belonging to a higher order of the regulatory hierarchy. Indeed, the nuclear-cytosol androgen-receptor protein has been found to have all the attributes of being the master regulatory gene product of the secondary (extragonadal) sex-determining mechanism of mammals.

Accordingly, the thought that this receptor protein might be the product specified by the X-linked Tfm locus entered our minds almost immediately after beginning our systematic study of Tfm/Y mice. During 1970 and 1971, steroid receptor studies were still in their infancy. Many a protein that demonstrated a relatively high binding affinity to androgens had been mistaken for the nuclear-cytosol receptor. In view of the naiveté of steroid receptor investigators of those years, it was extremely fortunate indeed that my first study on the nuclear-cytosol androgen receptor of affected Tfm/Y mice was done in cooperation with the late Gordon Tomkins, who had an extraordinarily sagacious mind, and his colleague Ulrich Gehring (GEHRING et al., 1971). On the mouse kidney, it was clearly shown that compared to +/Y males and +/+ females, Tfm/Y target cells were endowed with only 20% a s many androgen receptors (Fig. 33). The next published study on androgen-receptors of Tfm/Y mice promptly mistook a small 2 - 3S protein peculiar to mouse submaxillary salivary glands for androgen receptors, and a claim was made that Tfm/Y target cells were endowed with an above normal level of androgen receptors (WILSON and GOLDSTEIN, 1972).

Equally fortunate was the fact that a mutational deficiency of the nuclear-cytosol androgen-receptor protein that charaterized Tfm/Y mice was of the most easily recognizable type. One can easily imagine a few different kinds of much subtler mutations that can also render a mutated receptor functionless, for example, a failure by a mutated receptor to undergo a proper allosteric change to create the acceptor binding site in response to the act of androgen binding. Even today, I doubt if anyone can distinguish this ty pe of subtly altered mutant receptor from the wild-type receptor (AMRHEIN et al., 1976). Nevertheless, I must confess that during 1972 and 1973 I entertained a very grave doubt as to whether an observed deficiency of the nuclear-cytosol androgen-receptor protein was the real cause of the total androgen nonresponsiveness exhibited by Tfm/Y. My doubt was caused by the following two observations:

1. The binding affinity to 5α-dihydrotestosterone of the wild-type androgen-receptor protein appeared too low for it to function as the true regulatory protein. I now realize that the Kd of roughly 1.0×10^{-9} M for the above-noted androgen is proper for the assigned function of the androgen-receptor protein. Were it to be endowed with any higher binding affinity, by responding to the normal female testosterone concentration, it would inadvertently masculinize the female.

2. In the cytosol, there was an 80% difference in the androgen-receptor level between wild-type mice and Tfm/Y mice, as already noted. When the levels were compared on isolated target cell nuclei, however, the difference diminished to a mere 40% - 50% (GEHRING et al., 1971; DREWS et al., 1972). When the nuclear levels, retained after extensive KC1 extractions, were compared, the difference no longer existed. At the time, it was thought that the last category of tightest nuclear binding represented the functionally most important bindings between the acceptor binding sites on the target chromatin and androgen-bound receptor molecules. Of course, we now know that this type of nuclear binding study represents the last reliable part of the steroid-receptor research, and that the tightest binding appears to involve highly repetitious DNA, constituting the most dispensable fraction (the constitutive heterochromatin) of the mammalian genome.

As the search for an alternative candidate that might better fit the role of being the Tfm gene product failed, we resumed the study of the nuclear-cytosol androgen-receptor of the mouse. Meanwhile, a similar androgen-receptor deficiency was described in Tfm/Y rats (BARDIN et al., 1973) and in Tfm/Y women (KEENAN et al., 1974). Thus, the evidence in favor of the view that the nuclear-cytosol androgen-receptor protein is the master regulatory gene product specified by the X-linked Tfm locus became rather overwhelming. At this stage, what was ardently sought was any evidence that would prove a mutational alteration of the Tfm/Y androgen receptor-protein. At various times, Barbara Attardi and I felt that there existed a demonstrable difference between the wild-type and Tfm androgen-receptor proteins with regard either to relative binding affinities toward 5a-dihydrotestosterone and testosterone or to their isoelectric points. When these leads were pursued further, however, the apparent difference disappeared. The same apparently holds true in Tfm/Y rats and Tfm/Y women. Accordingly, the identy between the X-linked Tfm locus and the nuclear-cytosol androgen-receptor protein structural locus still remains an assumption.

Nevertheless, the assumption is supported by rather strong indirect evidence. Befitting its X-linkage, the body of Tfm/+ heterozygotes consists of androgen-nonresponsive Tfm clones and normally responsive wild-type + clones. In the mouse, the presence of these two clones has been demonstrated in the kidney (see

Fig. 26) as well as in male accessory reproductive organs of sex-reversed Tfm/+, Sxr/- males (see Fig. 28). Using cultured fibroblasts obtained from mothers of Tfm/Y women who therefore were obligatory Tfm/+ heterozygotes, Meyer et al., (1975) managed to separate two clones, one containing the wild-type level of androgen receptor and the other a very low mutant level. Thus, the manifestation of Tfm effects as well as the expression of androgen receptor is hemizygous, obeying the law of X-inactivation (LYON, 1961; BBEUTLER et al., 1962). In the mouse, whenever nuclear-cytosol androgen-receptor levels of corresponding organs were compared between wild-type males and females, on the one hand, and Tfm/Y on the other, exactly the same degreee of difference was observed in every instance (Fig. 33).

c) Two Tfm Gene Loci on the Mammalian X?

When several Tfm/Y women, presumably representing different, independently sustained mutations of the X-linked Tfm locus, were studied for their androgen receptors, a clear-cut deficiency as described in the original paper (KEENAN et al., 1974), was found only in about half of them. The other half wer endowed with apparently normal androgen receptors, based on their measurable properties (AMRHEIN et al., 1976). Provided that those of the second group were as androgen nonresponsive as the affected of the first type, the above finding *per* is still not disturbing. I have already noted that of several different types of mutations that can render mutated androgen-receptor proteins functionally defunct, our present technology permits us to identify only some of them as abnormal. What is needed here is a complementation test on somatic hybrids between the two types. If hybrids remain androgen nonresponsive, apparently normal androgen-receptor proteins possessed by affected individuals of the second type are indeed functionless. It is unforunate that even wild-type fibroblasts demonstrate no measurable androgen response. If the successful complementation test, done in the future, possibly on another cell type, proves that the androgen responsiveness is restored to somatic hybrids between the two types of Tfm/Y, I shall then entertain the possibility that the androgen receptor consists of two different subunits specified by two closely linked Tfm genes on the X, and that only one of the two subunits carries the androgen-binding site. It is well worth remembering that we thus far have identified the androgen, and all other steroid hormone-receptors, only through labeled steroids used as probes. The question of whether there is only one or, in fact, two X-linked genes for the regulation of the mammalian secondary sex-determining meachanism, however, is about as important as the question of whether the mammalian Y chromosome carries single or multiple copies of the testis-organizing H-Y gene, as discussed at the end of Part II. The point of this book is that the mammalian sex-determining mechanism consists of two independent regulatory hierarchies and that each is placed under the control of essentially one master regulatory gene product.

References

AKRAM, H., WENIGER, J-P.: Feminization en culture *in vitro* du testicule embryonaire de poulet par le testicule embryonaire de veau. Arch. Anat. Micro. Morphol. Exp. *57*, 369-378 (1968)

ALLISON, J. E., STANLEY, A. J., GUMBRECK, L. G.: Male pseudohermaphroditic rats. Anat. Rec. *153*, 85-86 (1965)

AMRHEIM, J. A., MEYER, W. J. IIIRD., JONES, H. W. JR., MIGEON, C. J.:
Androgen insensitivities in man: Evidence for genetic heterogeniety. Proc. Nate. Acad. Sci. USA *73*, 891-894 (1976)

ANON (anonimous).: Effects of sexual activity on beard growth of man. Nature London *226*, 869-870 (1970)

ARNASSON, U.: The role of chromosomal rearrangements in mammalian speciation with special reference to Cetacea and Pinnipedia. Hereditas *70*, 113-124 (1972)

ATTARDI, B., OHNO, S.: Cytosol androgen-receptor from kidney of normal and testicular feminized (Tfm) mice. Cell *2*, 205-212 (1974)

ATTARDI, B., GELLER, N., OHNO, S.: Androgen and estrogen receptors in brain cytosol from male, female and testicular feminized (Tfm/Y) mice. Endocrinology *98*, 864-874 (1976)

ATTARDI, B., OHNO, S.: Androgen and estrogen receptors in the developing mouse brain. Endocrinology *99*, 1279-1290 (1976)

ATTARDI, B., RUOSLAHTI, E.: Foetoneonatal oestradiol-binding protein in mouse brain cytosol is *a*-foetoprotein. Nature (London) *263*, 685-687 (1976)

BARDIN, C.W., BULLOCK, L. P., SHERINS, R. J., MOWSZOVICZ, I. BLACKBURN, W. R.: Androgen metabolism and mechanism of action in male pseudohermaphroditism: A Study of testicular feminization. Recent Prog. Horm. Res. *29*, 65-105 (1973)

BASTOS, R. N., AVIV, H.: Globin RNA precursor molecules; biosynthesis and processing in erythroid cells. Cell *11*, 641-650 (1977)

BAULIEU, E-E., JUNG, I.: A prostatic cytosol receptor. Biochem. Biophys. Res. Commun. *38*, 599-606 (1970)

BENIRSCHKE, K., BROWNHILL, L. E.: Heterosexual cells in testes of chimeric marmoset monkeys. Cytogenetics *2*, 331-341 (1963)

BENNETT, D., BOYSE, E. A., LYON, M. F., MATHIESON, B. J., SCHEID, M., YANAGISAWA, K.: Expression of H-Y (male) antigen in phenotypically female Tfm/Y mice. Nature (London) *257*, 236-238 (1975)

BENNETT, D., BOYSE, E. A., MATHIESON, B. J., SCHEID, M., WACHTEL, S. S., YANAGISAWA, K., CATTANACH, B. M.: Serological evidence for H-Y antigen in Sxr-XX sex-reversed phenotypic males. Nature (London) *265*, 255-257 (1977)

BENOIT, J.: Transformation experimentale du sexe ovariotomie precoce chez la poule domestique. C. R. Acad. Sci. (Paris) *177*, 1074-1077 (1923)

BERNHARDI, F. von.: Germany and The Next War (Transl. by Powles, A. H.). London: E. Arnold, 1914

BERTHEZENE, F., FOREST, M. G., GRIMAUD, J. A., CLAUSTRAT, B., MORNEX, R., Leydig cell agenesis: a cas of male pseudohermaphroditism. New. Engl. J. Med. *295*, 1112-1125 (1976)

BERTRAM, B. C. R.: The social system of lions. Sci. Am. *232*, 54-65 (1975)

BEUTLER, E., YEH, M., FAIRBANKS, V. F.: The normal human female as a mosaic of X-chromosome activity: Studies using the gene for G-6-PD deficiency as a marker. Proc. Nate. Acad. Sci. USA *48*, 9-16 (1962)

BEUTLER, B., NAGAI, Y., OHNO, S., KLEIN, G., SHAPIRO, I.: The HLA dependent expression of testis-organizing H-Y antigen by human male cells. Cell *13*, 509-513 (1978)

BIDLINGMAIER, F., KNORR, D., NEUMANN, F.: Inhibition of masculine differentiation in male offspring of rabbits actively immunized against testosterone before pregnance. Nature (London) *266*, 647-648 (1977)

BILLINGHAM, R. E., SILVERS, W. K.: Inbred animals and tissue transplantation immunity. Transplant. Bull. *6*, 339-406 (1959)

BLANK, K. J., LILLY, F.: Evidence for an H-2/viral protein complex on the cell surface as the basis of H-2 restriction of cytotoxicity. Nature (London) *269*, 808-809 (1977)

BOTTURA, C., FERRARI, I.: Male pseudohermaphroditism with XO chromosomal constitution in bone marrow cells. Brit. Med. J. *2*, 1100-1101 (1962)

BOYSE, E. A., Old, L. J., STOCKERT, E.: An approach to the mapping of antigens on the cell surface. Proc. Nate. Acad. Sci. USA *60*, 886-893 (1968)

BRADEN, A. W. H.: T-locus in mice: Segregation distortion and sterility in the male. In: The Genetics of The Spermatozoon. Beatty, R. A., GLUECKSOHN-WAELSCH, S. (Eds.) Copenhagen: Bogtrykkeriet Forum, 1972, pp. 289-305

BREEUWSMA, A. J.: Studies on Intersexuality in Pigs. Rotterdam: Drukkerij Bronder-Offset N. V. 1970

BROWN, D. D., DAWID, I. B.: Specific gene amplification in oöcytes. Science *160*, 272-280 (1968)

BRUCHOVSKY, N., WILSON, J. D.: Conversion of testosterone to $5a$-androstan-17β-01-3-one by rat prostates in vivo and in vitro. J. Biol. Chem. *243*; 2012-2019 (1968a)

BRUCHOVSKY, N., WILSON, J. D.: The intranuclear binding of testosterone and $5a$-androstan-17β-01-3-one by rat prostate. J. Biol. Chem. *243*, 5953-5960 (1968b)

BUBBERS, J. E. LILLY, F.: Selective incorporation of H-2 antigenic determinants into Friend virus particles. Nature (London) *266*, 458-459 (1977)

BULLOCK, L. P., BARDIN, C. W., OHNO, S.: The androgen insensitive mouse: Absence of intracellular androgen retention in the kidney. Biochem. Biophys. Res. Commun. *44*, 1537-1543 (1971)

BULLOCK, L. P., BARDIN, C. W.: The presence of estrogen receptor in kidneys from normal and androgen (insensitive Tfm/Y mice. Endocrinology *97*, 1106-1111 (1975)

CASTRO-SIERRA, E., WOLF, U.: Studies on the male meiosis of *Ellobius lutescens* Th. Cytogenetics *7*, 241-248 (1968)

CATTANACH, B. M., IDDON, C. A., CHARLTON, H. M., CHIAPPA, S. A., FINK, G.: Gonadotrop in-releasing hormone deficiency in a mutant mouse with hypogonadism. Nature (London) *269*, 338-340 (1977)

CATTANACH, B. M., POLLARD, C. E., HAWKES, S. G.: Sex-reversed mice: XX and XO males. Cytogenetics *10*, 318-327 (1971)

CHAPELLE, A. DE LA.: Nature and origin of males with XX sex chromosomes. Am. J. Hum. Genet. *24*, 71-105 (1972)

CICCARESE, S., OHNO, S.: Two plasma membrane antigens of testicular Sertoli cells and H-2 restricted versus unrestricted lysis by female T-cells. Cell *13*, 643-650 (1978)

COOKE, H.: Repeated sequence specific to human males. Nature (London) *262*, 182-186 (1976)

CRESSWELL, P., SPRINGER, R., STROMINGER, J. L., TURNER, M. J., GREY, H. M., KUBO, R. T.: Immunological identity of the small subunit of the HLA antigens as β_2-microglobulin and its turn over on the cell membrane. Proc. Nate. Acad. Sci. USA *71*, 2123-2127 (1974)

CROW, J. F., KIMURA, M.: An Introduction to Population Genetics Theory. New York: Harper and Row, 1970

CULLEN, S. E., BERNOCO, D., CARBONARA, A. O., JACOT-GUILLAERMOD, H., TRINCHIERI, G., CEPPELLINI, R.: Fate of HLA antigens and antibodies at the lymphocyte surface. Transplant Proc. *4*, 1835-1847 (1973)

CUNHA, R.: Tissue interactions between epithelium and mesenchyme of urogenital and integumental origin. Anat. Rec. *172*, 529-542 (1972)

CUNNINGHAM, B. A.: The structure and function of histocompatibility antigens. Sci. Am. *237*, 96-107 (1977)

CURMAN, B., ÖSTBERG, L., SANDBERG, L., MALMHEDEN-ERICSSON, I., RASK, L., PETERSON, P. A.: H-2 linked Ss protein is C4 component of complement. Nature (London) *258*, 243-245 (1975)

CUTLER, R. G.: Redundancy of information content in the genome of mammalian species as a protective mechanism determining aging rate. Mech. Ageing Dev. *2*; 381-408 (1973/74)

CUTLER, R. G.: Evolution of human longevity and the genetic complexity governing ageing rate. Proc. Nate. Acad. Sci. USA *72*, 4664-4668 (1974)

DARWIN, C.: The Descent of Man and Selection in Relation to Sex. London.: J. Murray, 1871, Vol. II.

DAWKINS, R.: The Selfish Gene. Oxford-London-New York: Oxford Univ. Press, 1976

DELANGE, R.L., FAMBROUGH, D.M.: Identical COOH-terminal sequences of arginine-rich histone from calf and pea. Fed. Proc. Am. Soc. Expt. Biol. *27*, 392 (1968)

DOFUKU, R., TETTENBORN, U., OHNO, S.: Testosterone "regulon" in the mouse kidney. Nature New Biol. *232*, 5-7 (1971a)

DOFUKU, R., TETTENBORN, U., OHNO, S.: Further characterization of Os mutation of β-gluculonidase locus. Nature New Biol. *234*, 259-261 (1971b)

DREWS, U., ITAKURA, H., DOFUKU, R., TETTENBORN, U., OHNO, S.: Nuclear DHT-receptors in Tfm/Y kidney cell. Nature New Biol. *238*, 216-217 (1972)

DREWS, U., BLECHER, S.R., OWEN, D.A., OHNO, S.: Genetically directed preferential X-inactivation seen in mice. Cell *1*, 3-8 (1974)

DREWS, U., DREWS, U.: Metabolic cooperation between Tfm and wild-type cells in mosaic mice after induction of DNA synthesis. Cell *6*, 475-479 (1975)

EICHWALD, E.J., SILMSER, C. R.: Communication. Transplant. Bull. *2*, 148-149 (1955)

EVANS, E. P., FORD, C.E., LYON, M.F.: Direct evidence of the capacity of XY germ cells in the mouse to become an oöcyte. Nature (London) *267*, 430-431 (1977)

FELLOUS, M., GÜNTHER, E., KEMLER, R., WIELS, J., BERGER, R., GUENET, J. L., JAKOB, H., JACOB, F.: Association of the H-Y male antigen with β_2-microglobulin on human lymphoid and differentiated mouse teratocarcinoma cells. J. Exp. Med. *148*, 58-76 (1978)

FERGUSSON-SMITH, M. A.: X-Y chromosome interchange in the aetiology of true hermaphroditism and of XX Klinefelter's syndrome Lancet, 475-476 (1966)

FISHMAN, W. H.: β-glucuronidase and the action of steroid hormones. Ann. N. Y. Acad. Sci. *54*, 548-557 (1951)

FLECHER, T.J., SHORT, R. V.: Restoration of libido in castrated red deer stag (Cervus elephus) with oestradiol-17β. Nature London *248*, 616-618 (1974)

FORD, C. E., EVANS, E. P.: Cytogenetic observation on XX/XY chimaeras and a reassessment of the evidence for germ cell chimaeras in heterosexual twin cattle and marmosets. J. Reprod. Fertil. *49*, 25-33 (1977)

FRACCARO, M., LINDSTEN, J.: The nature, origin and genetic implications of structural abnormalities of the sex chromosomes in man. In: Cytogenetics of Cells in Culture. Harris, R. J. C. *(Ed.)* New York: Academic Press 1964

FREDGA, K.: Unusual sex chromosome inheritance in mammals. Philos. Trans. R. Soc. Lond. B*259*, 15-39 (1970)

FREDGA, K., GROPP, A., WINKING, H., FRANK, F.: Fertile XX- and XY-type females in the wood lemming (Myopeus schisticolor). Nature London *261*, 255-257 (1976)

FRENCH, F. S., RITZEN, E. M.: A high affinity androgen-binding protein (ABP) in rat testis: Evidence for secretion into efferent duct fluid andabsorption by epididymis. Endocrinology *93*, 88-95 (1973)

GARDNER, B. T., GARDNER, R. A.: Evidence for sentence constructions in the early utterances of child and chimpanzee. J. Exp. Psychol. *104*, 244-261 (1975)

GEHRING, U., TOMKINS, G.M., OHNO, S.: Effect of the androgen insensitivity mutation on a cytoplasmic receptor for dihydrotestosterone. Nature New Biol. *232*, 106-107 (1971)

GEIB, R., GOLDBERG, E. H., KLEIN, J.: Membrane-bound H-2 and H-Y antigens move independently of each other. Nature London *270*, 352-354 (1977)

GHETIE, U., NILSSON, K., SJÖQUIST, J.: Detection and quantitation of lgG on the surface of human lymphoid cells by rosette formation with protein-A coated red blood cells. Eur. J. Immunol. *4*, 500-505 (1974)

GILMORE, D.G.: Histocompatibility antigen in the heterogametic sex in the chicken. Transplantation *5*, 609-709 (1967)

GOLDBERG, E. H., BOYSE, E. A., BENNETT, D., SCHEID, M., CARSWELL, E. A.: Serological demonstration of H-Y (male) antigen on mouse sperm. Nature London *232*, 378-380 (1971)

GOLDBERG, E. H., BOYSE, E. A., SCHEID, M., BENNETT, D.: Production of H-Y antibody by female mice that fail to reject male skin. Nature New Biol. *238*, 55-57 (1972)

GOLDSTEIN, J. L., WILSON, J. D.: Studies on the pathogenesis of the pseudohermaphroditism in the mouse with testicular feminization. J. Clin. Invest. *51*, 1647-1655 (1972)

GOODFELLOW, P. N., JONES, E. A., HEYNINGEN, V. van., SOLOMON, E., BOBROW, M., MIGGIANO, V., BODMER, W. F.: β_2-microglobulin gene ist on chromosome 15 and not in the HLA region. Nature (London) *254*, 267-269 (1975)

GORDON, R. D., SIMPSON, E., SAMELSON, L. E.: *In vitro* cell mediated immune response to the male specific (H-Y) antigen in mice. J. Exp. Med. *142*, 1108-1120 (1975)

GORDON, R. D., MATHIESON, B. J., SAMELSON, L. E., BOYSE, E. A., SIMPSON, E.: The effect of allogeneic presentation on H-Y graft survival and *in vitro* cell mediated responses to H-Y antigen. J. Exp. Med. *144*, 810-826 (1976)

GORDON, R. D., SAMELSON, L. E., SIMPSON, E.: Selective response to H-Y antigen by F1 female mice sensitized to F1 male cells. J. Exp. Med. *146*, 606-610 (1977)

GORSKI, R. A.: Localization and sexual differentiation of the nervous structures which regulate ovulation. J. Reprod. Fertil. (Suppl. 1) 67-88 (1966)

GROBSTEIN, C.: Mechanism of organogenetic tissue interaction. Natl. Cancer Inst. Monogr. *26*, 279-299 (1967)

GROPP, A., OHNO, S.: The presence of a common embryonic blastema for ovarian and testicular parenchymal (follicular, interstitial and tubular) cells in cattle (*Bos taurus*). Z. Zellforsch. *74*, 505-528 (1966)

GROPP, A., WINKING, H., FRANK, F., NOACK, G., FREDGA, K.: Sex-chromosome aberrations in wood lemmings (*Myopus schisticolor*). Cytogenet. Cell Genet. *17*, 343-358 (1976)

GUSTAFSSON, J-A., STEINBERG, A.: Specificity of neonatal, androgen-induced imprinting of hepatic steroid metabolism in rats. Science *191*, 203-204 (1976)

HAMERTON, J. L.: Significance of sex chromosome derived heterochromatin in mammals. Nature (London) *219*, 910-913 (1968)

HAMERTON, J. L., DICKSON, J. M., POLLARD, C. E., GRIEVES, S. A., SHORT, R. V.: Genetic intersexuality in goats. J. Reprod. Fertil. (Suppl. 7) 25-51 (1969)

HAMPTON, S. M. H.: Gametogenesis in Marmosets: Ph. D. thesis. Houston, Univ. Texas, 1970

HANSEN, T. H., SHREFFLER, D. C.: Characterization of a constitutive variant of the murine serum protein allotype, *Slp*. J. Immunol. *117*, 1507-1513 (1976)

HANSSON, V., TRIGSTAD, O., FRENCH, F. S., MCLEARN, W. S., SMITH, A. A. TINDALL, D. J., WEDDINGTON, S. C., PETRUSZ, P., NAYFEH, S. N., RITZEN, E. M.: Androgen transport and receptor mechanisms in testes and epididymis. Nature (London) *250*, 387-391 (1974)

HARRIS, G. W.: Sex hormones, brain development and brain function. Endocrinology *75*, 627-648 (1964)

HAUSCHKA, T. S., GRINNELL, S. T., MEAGHER, M., AMOS, D. B.: Sex-linked incompatibility of male skin and primary tumors transplanted to isologous female mice. In: Genetics and Cancer. Austin: Univ. Texas Press, 1959 pp. 271-293

HAYMAN, D. L., MARTIN, P. G.: Sex chromosome mosaicism in marsupial genera, *Isoodon* and *Perameles*. Genetics *52*, 1201-1206 (1965)

HENNING, R., SCHRADER, J. W. EDELMANN, G. M.: Antiviral antibodies inhibit the lysis of tumor cells by anti-H-2 sera. Nature (London) *263*, 689-691 (1976)

HILDEMAN, W. H., MORGAN, M. FRAUTNICK, L.: Immunogenetic components of weaker histoincompatibility systems in mice. Transplant. Proc. *2*, 24-39 (1970)

HOZUMI, N., TONEGAWA, S.: Evidence for somatic rearrangement of immuno-globulin genes coding for variable and constant regions. Proc. Nate. Acad. Sci. USA *73*, 3628-3632 (1976)

HSU, T. C., BENIRSCHKE K.: An Atlas of Mammalian Chromosomes. Folio 88. Berlin-Heidelberg-New York: Springer, 1968, Vol. III

IMPERATO-MCGINLEY, J., GUERRERO, L., GAUTHIER, T. PETERSON, R. E.: Steroid 5*a*-reductase deficiency in man: An inherited form of male pseudohermaphroditism. Science *186*, 1213-1215 (1974)

INHORN, S. L., OPITZ, J. M.: abnormalities of sex development. In: Endocrine Pathology. Bloodworth, J. M. B. Jr. (Ed.) Baltimore: Williams and Wilkins, 1968, pp. 529-606

ITAKURA, H., OHNO, S.: The effect of the mouse X-linked testicular feminization mutation on the hypothalamo-pituitary axis. 1. Paradoxical effect of testosterone upon pituitary gonadotrophs. Clin. Genet. *4*, 91-97 (1973)

JACOBS, P. A., STRONG, J. A.: A case of human intersexuality having a possible XXY sex determining mechanism. Nature (London) *183*, 302-303 (1959)

JERNE , N. K.: Somatic generation of immune recognition. Europ. J. Immunol. *1*, 1-9 (1971)

JIRASEK, J. E.: Morphogenesis of the genital system in the human. In: Morphogenesis and Malformation of the Genital System. The National Foundation Birth Defects: Original Article Series, Blandau R. J., Bergsma D. (Eds.) New York: Allan R. Liss, 1977, Vol. VIII, pp. 13-19

JONES, R. B., NOWELL, N. W.: Effects of androgen on the aversive properties of male mouse urine. J. Endocrinol. *60*, 19-25 (1974)

JOSSO, N., PICARD, J-Y., TRAN, D.: The anti-Müllerian hormone. In: Morphogenesis and Malformation of The Genital System, The National Foundation, Birth Defects; Original Article Series. Blandau, R. J. and Bergsma, D. ed.). New York: Alan R. Liss, 1977 Vol. XIII, pp. 59-84

JOST, A.: Sur le effets de la castration précoce de l'embryon mâle de lapin. C. R. Soc. Biol. (Paris). *141*, 126-129 (1947a)

JOST, A.: Action de la testostérone sur l'embryon mâle castré de lapin. C. R. Soc. Biol. (Paris). *141*, 275-278 (1947b)

JOST, A., PERCHELLET, J. P., PREPIN, J., VIGIER, B.: The prenatal development of bovine freemartins. In: Intersexuality in The Animal Kingdom. Reinboth, R., (Ed.). Berlin-Heidelberg-New York: Springer, 1975, pp. 392-406

JOST, A., PREPIN, J., VIGIER, B.: Hormones in the morphogenesis of the genital system. In: Morphogenesis and Malformation of The Genital System, The National Foundation Birth Defects: Original Article Series. New York: Alan R. Liss, 1977, Vol. XIII, pp. 85-97

JULIUS, M. H., SIMPSON, E., HERZENBERG, L. A.: A rapid method for the isolation of functional thymus-derived murine lymphocytes. Eur. J. Immunol. *3*, 645-649 (1973)

JUNG, I., BAULIEU, E-E.: Testosterone cytosol "receptor" in the rat levator ani muscle. Nature New Biol. *237*, 24-26 (1972)

JUNG-TESTAS, I., BAYARD, F., BAULIEU, E-E.: Two sex steroid receptors in mouse fibroblasts in culture. Nature (London) *259*, 136-138 (1976)

KALLMAN, K. D.: Genetics of tissue transplantation in teleostei. Transplant. Proc. *2*, 263-271 (1970)

KAN, J.D., MACKINNON, P. C. B. OHNO, S., YOUNGLAI, E. V.: The restoration of androgen sensitivity in the hypothalamo-pituitary axis of the testicular feminized (Tfm/Y) mouse by a "position effect". J. Physiol. *242*, 103 (1975)

KANAGAWA,, H., MURAMOTO, J., KAWATA, K., ISHIKAWA, T.: Chromosome studies in heterosexual twins in cattle. 1. Sex chromosome chimaerism. Jpn. J. Vet. Res. *13*, 33-41 (1965)

KASDAN, R., NANKIN, H. R., TROEN, R., WALD, N., PAN, S., YANAIHARA, T.: Paternal transmission of maleness in XX human beings. New. Engl. J. Med. *288*, 539-545 (1973)

KATONGOLE, C. B., NAFTOLIN, F., SHORT, R. V.: Relationship between blood levels of luteinizing hormone and testosterone in bulls, and the effect of sexual stimulation. J. Endocrinol. *50*, 457-466 (1971)

KEENAN, B. S., MEYER, W. J. IIIrd., HADJIAN, A. J., JONES, H. W. Jr., MIGEON, C. J.: Syndrome of androgen insensitivity in man: Absence of 5*a*-dihydro- testosterone binding protein in skin fibroblasts. J. Clin. Endocrinol. Metab. *38*, 1143-1146 (1974)

KELLER, K., TANDLER, J.: Über das Verhalten der Eihäute bei Zwillingsträchtigkeit des Rindes. Wien. Tierärztl. Monatsschr. *3*, 513-527 (1917)

KING, M. C., WILSON, A. C.: Evolution at two levels in human and Chimpanzees. Science *188*, 107-116 (1975)

KLEIN, J.: The Mouse Histocompatibility-2 Complex. Berlin-Heidelberg-New York: Springer, 1975

KLEIN, G., TERASAKI, P., BILLING, R., HONIG, R., JONDAL, M., ROSEN, A., ZEUTHEN, J., CLEMENTS, G.: Somatic cell hybrids between human lymphoma lines. III. Surface markers. Int. J. Cancer *19*, 66-76 (1977)

KOO, G. C., STACKPOLE, C. W., BOYSE, E. A., HÄMMERLING, U., LARDIS, M.: Topographical location of H-Y antigen on mouse spermatozoa by immunoelectromicroscopy. Proc. Natl. Acad. Sci. USA *70*, 1502-1507 (1973)

KRATOCHWIL, K., SCHWARTZ, P.: Tissue interaction in androgen response of embryonic mammary rudiment of mouse: Identification of target tissue for testosterone. Proc. Natl. Acad. Sci. USA. *73*, 4041-4044 (1976)

KRCO, C. J., GOLDBERG, E. H.: H-Y (male) antigen: Detection on 8-cell embryos. Science *193*, 1134-1135 (1976)

LACHMAN, P. J., GRENNAN, D., MARTIN, A., DEMANT, P.: Identification of Ss protein as murine C4. Nature (London) *258*, 242-243 (1975)

LAWICK-GOODALL, H. van., PAWICK-GOODALL, J. van.: Innocent Killers. New York: Ballantine Books, 1970

LENZ, W.: Persistenz des Oviduktes beim Mann (*Pseudohermaphroditismus masculinus internus, tubular hermaphroditismus*). Humangenetik *3*, 390-401 (1954)

LEVI-MONTALCINI, R., ANGELETTI, P. U.: Growth control of the sympathetic system by a specific protein factor. Q. Rev. Biol. *36*, 99-108 (1961)

LIAO, S., LIANG, T., TYMOCZKO, J. L.: Ribonucleoprotein binding of steroid-"receptor" complexes. Nature New Biol. *241*, 211-212 (1973)

LIFSCHITZ, E.: XX-chromosome inactivation: An essential feature of normal spermiogenesis. In: The Genetics of The Spermatozoon. Beatty, R. A., Gluecksohn-Waelsch, S. (Eds.) Copenhagen: Bogtrykkeriet Forum, 1972, pp. 223-232

LILLIE, F. R.: The free-martin; a study of the action of sex hormones in the foetal life of cattle. J. Exp. Zool. *23*, 371-422 (1917)

LYAPNOVA, E. A., VORONTSOV, N. N., ZAKARIAN, G. G.: Zygotic motality in *Ellobius lutescens* (*Rodentia, Microtinae*). Experientia *31*, 417 (1975)

LYON, M. F.: Gene action in the X-chromosome of the mouse (*Mus musculus* L.). Nature (London) *190*, 372-373 (1961)

LYON, M. F., HAWKES, S. G.: An X-linked gene for testicular feminization of the mouse. Nature (London) *227*, 1217-1219 (1970)

LYON, M. F., HENDRY, I., SHORT, R. V.: The submaxillary salivary glands as test organs for response to androgen in mice with testicular feminization. J. Endocrinol. *58*, 357-362 (1973)

LYON, M. F., GLENISTER, P. H. LAMOREUX, M. L.: Normal spermatozoa from androgen-resistant germ cells of chimaeric mice and the role of androgen in spermatogenesis. Nature (London) *258*, 620-622 (1975)

LUTZ, H., LUTZ-OSTERTAG, Y.: Etude d'un freemary tin chez le oiseaux. Arch. Anat. Microsc. Morphd. Exp. *47*, 205-217 (1958)

MAINWARING, W. I. P.: A soluble androgen receptor in the cytoplasma of rat prostate. J. Endocrinol. *45*, 531-541 (1969)

MAINWARING, W. I. P., ANGAN, F. R.: A study of the androgen-receptors in a variety of androgen-sensitive tissues. J. Endocrinol. *59*, 121-139 (1973)

MANN, T.: Advances in male reproductive physiology. Fertil. Steril. *23*, 699-707 (1972)

McDONALD, P. G., DOUGHTY, C.: Effect of neonatal administration of different androgens in the female rat: Correlation between aromatization and the induction of sterilization. J. Endrocinol. *61*, 1025-1036 (1974)

McEWAN, B. S., PLAPINGER, L., CHAPTAL, C., GERLACH, J., WALLACE, G.: Role of fetoneonatal estrogen binding proteins in the association of estrogen with neonatal brain cell nuclear receptors. Brain Res. *96*, 400-406 (1975)

Mc KUSICK, V. A., RUDDLE, F. H.: The status of the gene map of the human chromosomes. Science *196*, 390-405 (1977)

Mc LAREN, A.: Mammalian Chimaeras. Development and Cell Biology 4. Cambridge-London-New York-Melbourne: Cambridge Univ. Press, 1976

Mc LAUGHLIN, P. J., DAYHOFF, M. O.: Atlas of Protein Sequence and Structure. Silver springs (Maryland): National Biomedical Research Foundation, 1969

MARSHALL, J. R., HAMMOND, C. B., ROSS., G. T., JACOBSON, A., RAYFORD, , P., ODELL, W. D.: Plasma and urinary chorionic gonadotropin during early human pregnancy. Obstet. Gynecol. *32*, 760-764 (1968)

MATTHEY, R.: Un nouveau type de determination chromosomique du sexe chez le mammiferes *Ellobius lutescens* Th. et *Microtus (Chilotus) oregoni* Bchm, (murides-microtines). Experientia *14*, 240-241 (1958)

MATTHEY, R.: Etude sur les chromosomes d'*Ellobius lutescens* Th. (*Mammalia-Muridae-Microtinae*). II. Informations complementaires sur les divisions meiotiques. Rev. Suisse Zool. *71*, 401-410 (1964)

MAZA, L. M. de la., SAWYER, J. R.: The G and Q banding pattern of *Ellobius lutescens*. A unique case of sex determination in mammals. Canad. J. Genet.Cytol. *18*, 497-507 (1976)

MEYER, W. J. IIIRD., MIGEON, B. R., MIGEON, C. J.: A locus on human X-chromosome for dihydrotestosterone receptor and androgen insensitivity. Proc. Nate. Acad. Sci. USA. *72*, 1469-1472 (1975)

MICHEL, G. BAULIEU, E-E.: Androgen receptor in skeletal muscle. J. Endrocrinol. *65*, 31-32 (1974)

MIKAMO, K., WITSCHI, E.: Masculinization and breeding of WW *xenopus*. Experientia *20*, 622-624 (1964)

MILLER, R. A.: Spermatogenesis in a sex-reversed female and normal males of the domestic fowl, *Gallus domesticus*. Anat. Rec. *70*, 155-189 (1938)

MONEY, J.: Influence of hormones in sexual behavior. Ann. Rev. Med. *16*, 67-82 (1965)

MORILLO-CUCCI, G., GERMAN, J.: Males with a uterus and Fallopian tubes; a rare disorder of sexual development. In: The Endocrine System, The National Foundation Birth Defects: Original Article Series. Bergsma, D. (Ed.), New York, Alan R. Liss, 1971, Vol. VII, pp. 229-231

MORRIS, D.: The Naked Ape. London: Jonathan Cape, 1967

MORRIS, J. M.: The syndrome of testicular feminization in male pseudohermaphrodites. Am. J. Obstet. Gynecol. *654*, 1192-1211 (1953)

MOSCONA, A.: The development *in vitro* of chimaeric aggregates of dissociated embryonic chick and mouse cells. Proc. Nate. Acad. Sci. USA *43*, 184-189 (1957)

MUGFORD, R. A., NOWELL, N. W.: The aggression of male mice against androgenized females. Psychone. Sci. *20*, 191-192 (1970)

MÜLLER, U., ASCHONEIT, I., Zenzes, M. T., WOLF, U.: Binding studies of H-Y antigen in rat testes: Indication for a gonad specific receptor. Human Genetics. *43*, 151-157 (1978)

NAGAI, Y., OHNO, S.: Testis-determining H-Y antigen in X0 males of the mole vole (*Ellobius lutescens*). Cell *10*, 729-732 (1977)

NILSON, K., Erwin, P. E., WELSH, K. I.: Production of β_2-microglobulin by normal and malignant human cell lines and peripheral lymphocytes. Transplant. Rev. *21*, 53-84 (1974)

OHNO, S.: Sex Chromosomes and Sex-Linked Genes. Berlin-Heidelberg-New York: Springer 1967

OHNO, S.: An argument for the simplicity of mammalian regulatory systems: Single gene determination of male and female phenotypes. Nature (London) *234*, 134-138 (1971)

OHNO, S.: Animal Cytogenetics: Protochordata, Cyclostomata and Pices. Berlin-Stuttgart: Gebrüder Bornträger, 1974

OHNO, S.: The development of sexual reproduction. In: The Evolution of Reproduction, Reproduction in Mammals. Austin C. R. Short, R. V. (Eds) Cambridge-London-Melbourne: Cambridge Univ. Press, 1976a, Vol. VI, pp. 1-31

OHNO, S.: Secual differentiation and testosterone production. New Engl. J. Med. *295*, 1011-1012 (1976b)

OHNO, S.: Major regulatory genes for mammalian sexual development. Cell *7*, 315-321 (1976c)

OHNO, S.: The Y-linked H-Y antigen locus and the X-linked *Tfm* locus as major regulatory genes of the mammalian sex determining mechanism. J. Steroid Biochem. *8*, 585-592 (1977a)

OHNO S.: The original function of MHC antigens as the general plasma membrane anchorge sites of organogenesis-directing proteins. Immunol. Rev. *33*, 59-69 (1977b).

OHNO, S.: Testosterone and cellular response. In: Morphogenesis and Malformation of The Genital System. The National Foundation Birth Defects: Original Article Series, Blandau, R. J., Bergsma, D. (Eds). New York: Alan R. Liss, 1977c, Vol XIII, pp. 99-106

OHNO, S., ATKIN, N.B.: Comparative DNA values and chromosome complements of eight species of fishes. Chromosoma *18*, 455-466 (1966)

OHNO, S., BECAK, W., BECAK, M. L.: X-autosome ratio and the behavior pattern of individual X-chromosomes in placental mammals. Chromosoma *15*, 14-30 (1964)

OHNO, S., CHRISTIAN, L. C., WACHTEL, S. S., KOO., G. C.: Hormone-like role of H-Y antigen in bovine freemartin gonad. Nature (London) *261*, 597-598 (1976)

OHNO, S., CICCARESE, S., NAGAI, Y., WACHTEL, S. S.: H-Y antigen in testes of XX (BALB) /XY (C3H) chimaeric male mouse. Arch. Androl. *1*, 103-109 (1978a)

OHNO, S., DOFUKU, R., TETTENBORN, U.: More about X-linked testicular feminization of the mouse as a noninducible (is) mutation of a regulatory locus: $5a$-androstan-$3a$, 17β-diol as the true inducer of kidney alcohol dehydrogenase and β-glucuronidase. Clin. Genet. *2*, 128-140 (1971)

OHNO, S., GELLER, L. N., Kan, J. D.: The analysis of Lyon's hypothesis through preferential X-activation. Cell *1*, 175-181 (1974a)

OHNO, S., GELLER, L. N., YOUNGLAI, E. V.: *Tfm* mutation and masculinization versus feminization of the mouse central nervous system. Cell *3*, 235-242 (1974b)

OHNO S., GROPP, A.: Embryological basis for germ cell chimerism in mammals. Cytogenetics *4*, 251-261 (1965)

OHNO, S., JAINCHILL, J., STENIUS, C.: The creeping vole (*Microtus oregoni*) as a gonosomic mosaic: 1. The 0Y/XY chromosome constitution of the male.Cytogenetics *2*, 232-239 (1963)

OHNO, S., KAPLAN, W. D., KINOSITA, R.: Formation of the sex chromatin by a single X-chromosome in liver cells of *Rattus norvegicus*. Exp. Cell Res. *18*, 415-418 (1959)

OHNO, S. LYON, M. F.: X-lined testicular feminization in the mouse as a noninducible regulatory mutation of the Jacob-Monod type. Clin. Genet. *1*, 121-127 (1970)

OHNO, S., NAGAI, Y., CICCARESE, S.: Testicular cells lysostripped of H-Y antigen organize ovarian follicle-like aggregates. Cytogenet. Cell Genet. *20,* 351-364 (1978b)

OHNO, S., STENIUS, C., (1967) CHRISTIAN, L. C.: The X0 as the normal female of the creeping vole (*Microtus oregoni*). In: Chromosomes Today Darlington, C. D. Lewis, K. R. (Ed.) Edinburgh: Oliver and Boyd 1966, Vol. I, pp. 182-187

OHNO, S., TRUJILLO, J. M., STENIUS, C., CHRISTIAN, L. C., TEPLITZ, R.: Possible germ cell chimeras among newborn dizygotic twin calves (*Bos taurus*). Cytogenetics *1*, 258-265 (1962)

OVERZIER, C.: True hermaphroditism. In: Intersexuality. Overzier, C. Ed.). London-New York: Academic Press, 1963, pp. 192-234

PARDUE, M. L., Hsu, T. C.: Location of 18S and 28S ribosomal genes on the chromosomes of the Indian muntjac. J. Cell Biol. *64*, 251-254 (1975)

PEARSON, P. L., BOBROW, M., VOSA, C. G.: Technique for identifying Y chromosomes in human interphase nuclei. Nature (London) *226*, 78-80 (1970)

PELLINIEMI, L. J.: Ultrastructure of the early ovary and testis in pig embryos. Am. J. Anat. *144*, 89-111 (1975)

PELLINIEMI L. J., NIEMI, M.: Fine structure of human fetal testis. I. The interstitial tissue. Z. Zellforsch. *99*, 507-522 (1969)

PETERS, H.: Migration of gonocytes into the mammalian gonad and their differentiation. Philos. Trans. R. Soc. Lond. B259, 91-101 (1970)

PFAFF, D. W.: Steroid Sex hormones in the rat brain: Specificity of uptake and physiological effects. In: Steroid Hormones and Brain Function, Sawyer, C. H., Gorski, R. A. (Eds). Berkeley: Univ. California Press, 1971, pp. 103-116

POLANI, P. E.: Hormonal and clinical aspects of hermaphroditism and the testicular feminization syndrome in man. Philos. Trans. R. Soc. Lond. B259, 187-204 (1970)

PRADER, A.: Gonadendysgenesie und testikulare Feminisierung. Schweiz. Med. Wochenschr. *87*, 278-285 (1957)

RAYNAUD, A.: Effet des injections d'hormones sexuelles à la souris gravide, sur le dévelopment des ébauches de la glande mammaire des embryons. I. Action des substances androgénes. Ann. Endocrinol *8*, 248-253 (1947)

REED, K. C., OHNO, S.: Kinetic properties of human placental aromatase: Application of an assay measuring $^3H_20$ release from 1β, 2β, -^{3}H-androgens. J. Biol. Chem. *251*, 1625-1631 (1976)

REES, H.; DNA in higher plants. In: Evolution of Genetic Systems, Brookhaven Symposium in Biology., New York-London: Gordon and Breach, 1972, Vol. XXIII, pp. 394-418

REHDER, H.: Gonadentumoren bei Intersexualität. Gynäkologe *9*, 30-38 (1976)

REYES, F. I., BORODITSKY, R. S., WINTER, J. S. D., FAIMAN, C.: Studies on human sexual development. II. Fetal and maternal serum gonadotropin and sex steroid concentrations. J. Clin. Endocrinol. Metab. *38*, 612-617 (1974)

RITOSSA, F. M., ATWOOD, K. C., SPIEGELMAN, S.: A molecular explanation of the *bobbed* mutant of *Drosophila* as partial deficiencies of „ribosomal" DNA. Genetics *54*, 819-834 (1966)

ROUSEN-RUNGE, E. C.: Primordial germ cells and the spermatogonia. In: Congenital Malformation. New York: Inter. Medical Congress, 1964, pp. 32-35

RYAN, K. J., NAFTOLIN, F., REDDY, B., FLORES F., PETRO, A.: Estrogen formation in the brain. J. Obstet. Gynecol. *114*, 454-460 (1972)

SCHEID, M., BOYSE, E. A., CARSWELL, E. A., Old, L. J.: Serologically demonstrable alloantigens of mouse epidermal cells. J. Exp. Med. *135*, 938-955 (1972)

SCHENKEIN, I., LEVY, M., BUCKER, E. D., WILSON, J. D.: Immunological and enzymatic evidence for the absence of an esteroproteolytic enzyme (protease „D") in the submandibular gland of the *Tfm* mouse. Endocrinology *94*, 840-844, (1974)

SCHNEIDER, G, BARDIN, C. W.: Defective testicular testosterone synthesis by the pseudohermaphrodite rat: An abnormality of 17β-hydroxysteroid dehydrogenase. Endocrinology *87*, 864-873 (1970)

SCHRADER, J. W., CUNNINGHAM, B. A., EDELMANN, G. W.: Functional interaction of viral and histocompatibility antigens at tumor cell surface. Proc. Nate. Acad. Sci. USA. *75*, 5060-5070 (1975)

SCHULTZ, M., WILSON, J. D.: Virilization of the Wolffian duct in the rat fetus by various androgens. Endocrinology *94*, 979-987 (1974)

SELDEN, J. R., WACHTEL, S. S., KOO, G. C., HASKINS, M. E., PATTERSON, D. F.: Genetic basis of XX male syndrome and XX true hermaphroditism: Evidence in the dog. Science *201*, 644-646 (1978)

SHAPIRO, B. H., GOLDMANN, A. S., GUSTAFSSON, J-A.: Masculine-like hypothalamic-pituitary axis in the androgen-insensitive genetically male rat pseudohermaphrodite. Endocrinology *97*, 487-492 (1975)

SHORT, R. V.: The origin of species. In: The Evolution of Reproduction, Reproduction in Mammals, Cambridge-London-Melbourne: Cambridge Univ. Press, 1976, Vol. VI, pp. 110-148

SHORT, R. V., SMITH, J., MANN, T., EVANS, E. P., HALLET, J., FRYER, A., HAMERTON, J. L.: Cytogenetics and endocrine studies of a freemartin heifer and its bull co-twin. Cytogenetics *8*, 369-388 (1969)

SHREFFLER, D. C., OWEN, R. D.: A serologically detected variant in the mouse serum: Inheritance and association with the histocompatibility-2 locus. Genetics *48*, 9-25 (1963)

SIITERI R. K., WILSON, J. D.: Testosterone formation ane metabolism during male sexual differentiation in the human embryo. J. Clin. Endocrinology Metab *38*, 113-125 (1974)

SIMPSON, E., GORDON, R. D.: Responsiveness of H-Y antigen, Ir gene complementation and target cell specificity. Immunol. Rev. *35*, 59-75 (1977)

SINHA, Y. N., SALOCKS, C. G., LEWIS, U. J., VANDERLAAN, W. P.: Influence of nursing on the release of prolactin and GH in mice with high and low incidence of mammary tumors. Endocrinology *95*, 947-958 (1974)

STEINBERG, E., Hormonal control of mammalian spermatogenesis. Physiol. Rev. *51*, 1-22 (1971)

STEINITZ, B. G., GIANNINA, T., BUTLER, M., POPICK, F.: Dissociation of anabolic and androgenic properties of steroids by anti-anabolic and antiandrogenic agents in rats. Endocrinology *89*, 849-896 (1971)

STEINMULLER, D., EICHWALD, E. J.: A „subtractive" effect between H-2 and H-Y antigens. In: Symp. Immunogenetics of The H-2 System. (Liblice-Prague). Basel: Karger-Verlag, 1971, pp. 278-283

STERNBERG, W. H., BARCLAY, D. L. KLOEPFER, W. H.: Familial XY gonadal dysgenesis. New. Engl. J. Med. *278*, 695-702 (1968)

SWANK, R. T., PAIGEN, K., GANSCHOW, R. E.: Genetic control of glucuronidase induction in mice. J. Mol. Biol. *81*, 225-243 (1973)

TARKOWSKI, A. K.: Mouse chimaeras developed from fused eggs. Nature (London) *190*, 857-858 (1961)

TAYLOR, R. B., DUFFUS, P. H., RAFF, M. C., PETRIS, S. de.: Redistribution and pinocytosis of lymphocyte surface immunoglobulin antibody. Nature New Biol. *233*, 225-229 (1971)

TETTENBORN, U., DOFUKU, R., OHNO, S.: Noninducible phenotype exhibited by a proportion of female mice heterozygous for the X-linked testicular feminization mutation. Nature New Biol. *234*, 37-40 (1971)

TILGHMAN, S. M., CURTIS, P. J., TIEMEIER, D. C., LEDER, P., WEISSMANN, C.: The intervening sequence of a mouse β-globin gene is transcribed within the 15S β-globin *m*RNA precursor. Proc. Nat. Acad. Sci. USA *75*: 1309-1313 (1978)

TRAN, D., MEUSY-DESSOLLE, N., JOSSO, N.: Anti-müllerian hormone is a functional marker of foetal Sertoli cells. Nature (London) *269*, 411-412 (1977)

TOKUDA, S., ARRINGTON, T., GOLDBERG, E. H., RICHEY, J.: Simple technique for serological detection of H-Y antigen. Nature (London) *267*, 433-444 (1977)

TURKINGTON, R. W., BREW, K., VANAMAN, T. C., HILL, R. L.: The hormonal control of lactose synthetase in the developing mouse mammary gland. J. Biol. Chem. *243*, 3382-3391 (1968)

VANDEBERG, J. L., COOPER, D. W., Close, P.: Mammalian testis phosphoglycerate kinase. Nature New Biol. *243*, 48-50 (1973)

VIGIER, B., LOCATELLI, A., PREPIN, J., du Mesnil du Buisson, F., JOST, A.: Le premieres manifestation du „freemartinism" chez le faetus de veau ne dependent pas du chimerisme chromosomique XX/XY. C. R. Acad. Sci. (Paris) *285*, (Serie D) 1355-1358 (1976)

WACHTEL, S. S., KOO, G. C. BOYSE, E. A.: Evolutionary conservation of H-Y (male) antigen. Nature (London) *254*, 270-272 (1975a)

WACHTEL, S. S., OHNO, S., KOO, G. C., BOYSE, E. A.: Possible role of H-Y antigen in primary sex determination. Nature (London) *257*, 235-236 (1975b)

WACHTEL, S. S., KOO, G. C., BREG, W. R., ELIAS, S., BOYSE, E. A., MILLER, O.J.: Expression of H-Y antigen in human males with two Y chromosomes. Engl. J. Med. *293*, 1070-1072 (1975c)

WACHTEL, S. S., KOO, G. C., BREG, W. R., THALER, H. T., DILLARD, G. M., ROSENTHAL, I. M., DOSIK, H., GERALD, P. S., SAENGER, P., New, M., LIEBER, E., MILLER, O. J.: Serological detection of a Y-linked gene in XX males and XX true hermaphrodites. New. Engl. J. Med. *295*, 750-754 (1976a)

WACHTEL, S. S., KOO, G. C., OHNO, S., GROPP, A., DEI, V. G., TANTRAVAHI, R., MILLER, D. A., MILLER, O. J.: H-Y antigen and the origin of XY female wood lemmings (*Myopus schisticolor*). Nature (London) *264*, 638-639 (1976b)

WACHTEL, S. S., KOO, G. C., OHNO, S.: H-Y antigen and male development. In: The Testis in Normal and Infertile Men. TROEN, P., NANKIN, H. R. (Ed.) New York: Raven Press, 1977, pp. 35-43.

WEISS, E., HOFFMANN, R.: Eliminierung der XX-Zellen im Hoden heterosexueller Rinderzwillinge mit XX/XY chimerismus. Cytogenetics *8*, 68-73 (1969)

WELSHONS, W. J., RUSSELL, L. B.: The Y-chromosome as the bearer of male determining factors in the mouse. Proc. Nate. Acad. Sci. USA. *45*, 560-566 (1959)

WHITTEN, W. K.: Chromosomal basis for hermaphroditism in mice. In: The Developmental Biology of Reproduction (33rd Sym. Soc. Devel. Biol.), London-New York: Academic Press, 1975, pp. 189-205

WILSON, E. O.: Sociobiology: The New Synthesis. Cambridge (Mass.): Belknap, 1975

WILSON, J. D., GOLDSTEIN, J. L.: Evidence for increased cytoplasmic androgen binding in the submandibular gland of the mouse with testicular feminization. J. Biol. Chem. *247*, 7342-7348 (1972)

WITSCHI, E.: Migration of the germ cells of human embryos from the yolk sac to the primitive gonadal folds. Contrib. Embryol. Carneg. Inst. *32*, 67-80, (1948)

WITSCHI, E.: Genetic and postgentic sex determination. Experientia *14*, 274-278 (1960)

WURSTER, D. H., BENIRSCHKE, K.: Indian muntjac, *Muntjacus muntijak*; a deer with a low chromosome number. Science *168*, 1364-1365 (1970)

YAMAMOTO, T.: Progenies of sex-reversed males in the medaka, *Oryzias latipes*. J. Exp. Zool. *146*, 163-180 (1961)

ZENZES, M. T., WOLF, U., GÜNTHER, E., ENGEL, W.: Studies on the function of H-Y antigen: Dissociation and reorganization experiments on rat gonadal tissue. Cytogenet. Cell Genet. *20*, 365-372 (1978)

ZEUTHEN, J., FREIDRICH, U., ROSEN, A., KLEIN, E.: Structural abnormalities in chromosome 15 in cell lines with reduced expression of β_2-microglobulin. Immunogenetics. *4*, 567-580 (1977)

ZINKERNAGEL, R. M., DOHERTY, P. D.: Immunological surveillance against altered self components by sensitized T-lymphocytes in lymphocytic choriomeningitis. Nature (London) *251*, 547-549 (1974)

Subject Index

Other Volumes of Interest from this Series

Volume 10: W.I.P. Mainwaring

The Mechanism of Action on Androgens

1977. 12 figures, 17 tables. XI, 178 pages

ISBN 3-540-07941-6

Volume 9: R.E. Mancini

Immunologic Aspects of Testicular Function

1976. 36 figures, 8 tables. IX, 114 pages

ISBN 3-540-07496-1

Volume 8: E. Gurpide

Tracer Methods in Hormone Research

1975. 35 figures. XI, 188 pages

ISBN 3-540-07039-7

Volume 7: E.W. Horton

Prostaglandins

1972. 97 figures. XI, 197 pages

ISBN 3-540-95571-1

Volume 6: K. Federlin

Immunopathology of Insulin

Clinical and Experimental Studies

1971. 53 figures. XIII, 185 pages

ISBN 3-540-05408-1

Volume 5: J. Müller

Regulation of Aldosterone Biosynthesis

1971. 19 figures. VII, 137 pages

ISBN 3-540-05213-5

Volume 4: U. Westphal

Steroid - Protein Interactions

1971. 144 figures. XIII, 567 pages
ISBN 3-540-05312-3

Volume 3: F.G. Sulman

Hypothalamic Control of Lactation

In collaboration with M. Ben-David, A. Danon, S. Dikstein, Y. Givat, K. Khazen, J. Mishkinsky-Shani, I. Nir, C.P. Weller
1970. 58 figures. XII, 235 pages
ISBN 3-540-04973-8

Volume 2: K.B. Eik-Nes, E.C. Horning

Gas Phase Chromatography of Steroids

1968. 85 figures. XV, 382 pages
ISBN 3-540-04277-6

Volume 1: S. Ohno

Sex Chromosomes and Sex-Linked Genes

1967. 33 figures. X, 192 pages
ISBN 3-540-03934-1

In Preparation

Volume 12: J.D. Baxter, G.G. Rousseau

Glucocorticoid Hormone Action

1978. Approx. 178 figures, 58 tables. Approx. XVII, 550 pages
ISBN 3-540-08973-X

Volume 13: H.F. Deluca

Vitamin D – Metabolism and Function

1979. 14 figures. VI, approx. 100 pages
ISBN 3-540-09182-3

Springer-Verlag
Berlin
Heidelberg
New York